S0-BBN-837

UPDATED AND REVISED

FIGHT FAT & WIN!

How to Eat a Low-Fat Diet Without Changing Your Lifestyle

BY ELAINE MOQUETTE-MAGEE, M.P.H., R.D.

Fight Fat & Win! © 1994
by Elaine Moquette-Magee, M.P.H., R.D.

Library of Congress Cataloging-in-Publication Data

Moquette-Magee, Elaine.
Fight fat & win.
Includes index.
ISBN 1-56561-047-4
1. Low-fat diet. 2. Low-fat diet—Recipes. I. Title.
II. Title: Fight fat & win.
RM237.7.M67 1990 613.2'8 90-3532

Edited by: Patricia Richter
Photography: Jeff Natrop, Thoen Photography
Cover Design & Production: Wenda Johnson, Nancy Nies
Text Design: Claire Lewis
Typesetting/Production: Janet Hogge
Printed in the United States of America

10 9 8 7 6 5 4 3

Published by:

CHRONIMED/DCI Publishing
P.O. Box 47945
Minneapolis, MN 55447-9727

DEDICATION

Dedicated with love and respect to Jim Magee and Robert D. Frowein (Uncle Bob) whose lives were shortened by heart disease and cancer. Both deaths occurred during the years I was writing this book.

TABLE OF CONTENTS

ACKNOWLEDGMENTS

I want to thank my parents, Don and Nesly Moquette, who as far back as I can remember always told me, "You can do anything you set your mind to." Silly me . . . I actually believed them.

I thank God every day for giving me such a wonderful family (including my two sisters, Lynn Moquette O'Leary and Collette Moquette Ricks). It has made all the difference in my life. They've always been there for me with love and encouragement. And now, I can't believe how lucky I am. I have married into another exceptional family, the Magees. I love you all very much. Which brings me to my husband, Dennis.

The old saying goes, "Behind every successful man is a woman." Well, all I know is beside this particular nutrition writer is a very special and understanding man. And no matter how tense or frustrated I get before a big deadline, all I have to do is think of Dennis and I can't help but smile.

Now, for all the other wonderful people in my life. When a project like this one spans over three years of one's life, there ends up being countless people who contribute through either emotional or professional support. So this is my attempt to thank some of the people who contributed to the completion of this book.

I would like to thank Lori Kinser, who has not only been the best friend a woman could ever hope for, but who contributed to the book's conception and provided invaluable input throughout.

Several friends reviewed certain portions of the book for accuracy or practicality. Thank you all. Your time and suggestions meant a lot to me: Dr. Lorelei DiSogra, Patti Magee, Matthew Ricks, and Lynn Moquette O'Leary. Thanks also to Paul Rauber, Michael Fullerton, Russ Spencer, and my agent, Michael Snell, for their editing contributions.

FOREWORD

When I wrote this book over seven years ago, I had no idea eating a low-fat diet would gain so much momentum with media and health organizations so quickly. Consequently, more food companies have answered the resultant public plea by producing scores of new reduced fat and nonfat food products. In fact, it's a part-time job keeping up with it!

Even though several nutritionally enlightening years have gone by, *Fight Fat & Win* is still a great foundation and resource for those interested in eating a low-fat diet without changing their busy lifestyles. Gladly, though, we had to update the tables in the supermarket and fast-food chapters, since so many more reduced fat fast-food options and food products are available to us now.

During the past seven years, I have been madly experimenting with lowering fat from normally high-fat recipes, trying to perfect the art and science of cooking light. So we've added a section on "fat replacements" and "lightening up favorite holiday recipes." We also added 50 more recipes!

I still feel using the percentage of calories from fat is the most helpful way of assessing fat contribution to our overall diet, but I also now see the value of knowing the grams of fat per serving for a recipe, menu item, or food product as well. So I've taken the liberty of adding this extra bit of data to many of the tables in *Fight Fat & Win*.

To those of you who have been through some of these pages before, "Welcome back," and to new readers, happy reading and the best of health to you and your family.

Life in the Fat Lane

The stories you are about to hear could be true. (Then again they could be slightly exaggerated.)

The Working Parent

The buzzer goes off (sigh). . . you turn over, resting your head comfortably on your pillow, only to realize it's a work day and you have to get up. Between the time you take that first peaceful stretch and the time you race out the door, five minutes late, there seem to be a hundred things to do. You need to shower, get your children ready, iron a shirt, not to mention eating breakfast and packing lunches.

The Single Adult

You finally get off work. Your whole day has been a run-on sentence of appointments and phone calls. Now you have to rush to the automatic teller machine to get some cash so you can get to the dry cleaners before it closes at 5:30 to get your suit for tomorrow's meeting. (Somehow you lost the claim ticket so it takes them extra long to find that suit.) Then you barely make it to your 6 o'clock aerobics class and by the time you're showered, dressed, and on the road again, it's almost 8 P.M. Phew! Then . . .

- You could be meeting someone for a movie or coffee.
- You attend a night class or committee meeting.
- You're anxious to get home to watch your favorite sitcom—or you're just anxious to get home. (To play back the messages on the answering machine, maybe?)

On its own, being a "parent" or "having a career" keeps you busy enough, and some of us even manage to do both. Of course, there are other urgencies to squeeze into your schedule. Like exercise, family and friends, prayer or meditation, studying, and hobbies. Who doesn't consider themselves busy these days?

We might be busy, but aren't Americans today becoming more concerned about their health? Aren't we doing any better at the dinner table? Does the popular word "nutrition" simply represent vitamin supplements or alfalfa sprouts to most people, or has the concept of "improving our health through our diet (the foods we eat)" caught on—even a little?

According to preliminary findings of the U.S. National Health and Nutrition Examination Survey, apparently not. They found that the percentage of the population that is overweight today is greater than in the 1970s. And, more than 80 percent of adults recently surveyed failed the American Heart Association's National Nutrition Test.

In 1993, the American Dietetic Association surveyed 1,000 adults. While 79 percent of them rated nutrition as "at least moderately important," one third reported that how they actually eat is quite another matter.

This lapse in our national nutrition comes at a time when we are looking for changes in our health care system, but it seems that we are continuing to clog our arteries faster than we can find a way to guarantee health care for everyone at a reasonable cost. Recent information reinforces a 1988 article in the *New York Times* that discussed the results of a national telephone survey of 1,800 people ("What Americans Eat: Nutrition Can Wait, Survey Finds"). May I offer a few observations that might help us understand why we aren't eating as well as we think we are?

Observation #1.

One thing for sure, when it comes to nutrition as it relates to preventing disease and enhancing our total health, the interest is definitely there. More than half of the people surveyed said they had changed their eating habits in a major way in the past five years. Most of the women surveyed (60 percent) said they "Pay attention to salt at every meal." Slightly less than half said they were concerned about fats (46 percent) or sugar and sweets (42 percent). More than one fourth (31 percent) said they were interested in lowering cholesterol.

I don't know about you, but I think "paying attention to something" (or someone) at "every meal" is quite a commitment. And the fact that a large portion of the American population is willing to do this is . . . well, it's exciting!

The survey noted that what people said they paid attention to at every meal and what they actually did were quite different. But I don't totally blame the confused consumer for this little indiscretion. Certainly, all the nutrition and diet misinformation generated by food advertisers (trying to fit their products into the health food market) and pseudo-nutrition professionals (trying to sell their books) hasn't helped. Different health agencies and institutes handing out different diet guidelines (often on the same nutrient) telling us WHAT to do but not HOW to do it doesn't even come close to rescuing the consumer amidst all this confusion.

Observation #2.

People must also eat differently when eating out (and most of those people surveyed must have eaten out the day before). Supermarket sales have been showing that beef and egg consumption has persistently decreased since 1976, while fish and poultry sales are generally on the rise. From 1991 to 1992, the amount spent on beef, lamb, pork, and veal in grocery stores decreased 1.8 percent, while poultry sales increased 2.7%.

Observation #3.

I think there are some Americans eating "lighter meals" who frequently find themselves trapped in a "gourmet reward system." If they're "good" at a couple of meals, they later go for the rich desserts or fatty favorites—guilt free! Not that I'm into inflicting guilt, but I think people deserve to know how rich ice cream, flaky pastries, creamy entrees, deep-fried doodads, etc., day after day, influence daily totals of fat, saturated fat, cholesterol, and calories.

Observation #4.

America snacks in a big way. The younger generations seem to "graze" more than the older. But grazing (snacking) as an act isn't bad, it's what we graze on that usually makes it bad. For all generations, the number one snack, according to the *New York Times* survey, is sweets and ice cream. Chips, nuts, and popcorn come in second. When does America snack? Well, 14 percent said they snacked all day, and 33 percent said they snacked after dinner or before bed.

Observation #5.

Americans are indeed starting to get the message that excess fat, saturated fat, cholesterol, and sodium may be harmful to health. A recent Food Marketing Institute survey showed the same consumer trend the New York Times survey showed: People are becoming more concerned about specific nutrients rather than the concept of "nutrition" in general. They just don't know how to (and perhaps some just don't want to) translate these concerns into breakfast, lunch, or dinner decisions. Let's take a closer look at the way America is eating at breakfast, lunch, and dinner, and why we still have far to go.

Eating in the Fast Lane

When you think "typical American diet," what do you picture? Meat and potatoes? TV dinners? Guess again. In 1991, the average American spent $623 per person dining out, a majority of the money, according to the National Restaurant Association, was spent in fast food establishments. From 1991 to 1994, the annual growth rate in fast food sales has been 4.3 percent. In 1991, Americans spent almost $72 billion on fast food and by 1993, almost $81 billion.

Even TV dinners take too long to heat up in the oven, compared with the shelves of microwaveable gourmet and not-so-gourmet entrees available at supermarkets. And you can take your pick of fast food on your way to just about anywhere.

The 100-percent pure home-cooked meal (you know, the one demanding hours of preparation time) seems to have become extinct sometime between World War II and the sexual revolution of the '60s. It used to be accepted that mothers or housewives were the ones responsible for buying and making food for the family. But now that the big home-cooked meal is OUT and food in minutes is IN, food-buying decisions are up for grabs. It's every person for him or herself, and everyone becomes a "consumer." Kind of makes you feel liberated, doesn't it?

Every time we place a fast food or restaurant order, every time we pull a frozen entree from the freezer case or a can off the shelf, we are making a decision that affects our health. Problem is, the typical American let loose to make his or her own food choices isn't doing too well.

Let's find out the fatty truth about America's most loved meals, beginning with how some of us start our days.

❖ Mornings ❖

Typical Fast Food Choice
1 Sausage Biscuit (McDonalds)
582 calories, 1380 mg sodium, 61% calories from FAT

Typical Restaurant Choice
Ham and cheese (3 egg) omelette
3 slices bacon, hash browns
8 oz. whole milk
990 calories, 2061 mg sodium, 0.3 gm fiber
62% calories from FAT

❖ Lunches ❖

Typical Fast Food Choice

Big Mac, small fries, chocolate shake

1166 calories, 1419 mg sodium
41% calories from FAT

Typical Restaurant Choice

Chef salad

(1/4 cup creamy dressing, 2 cups lettuce with egg, ham, cheese, avocado, and tomato)

785 calories, 1422 mg sodium, 6 gm fiber
72% calories from FAT

(Do you carefully order the chef salad thinking you're not eating the calories and fat that usually comes with restaurant lunches? Try again.)

French Dip Sandwich

(6 oz. roast beef on a submarine roll, dipped in gravy)
1 cup potato salad
12 oz. whole milk

1628 calories, 1664 mg sodium, 4 gm fiber
53% calories from FAT

Typical Bag Lunch

Salami and cheese sandwich

(2 slices white bread, 5 slices dry salami, 2 oz. cheese, 2 teaspoons mayonnaise)

2 1/2 oz. bag of chips
12 oz. fruit soda

1059 calories, 1572 mg sodium, 55% calories from FAT

❖ Dinners ❖

Typical Fast Food Choice

1 Extra-Crispy Dinner (Kentucky Fried Chicken)

950 calories, 1915 mg sodium, 51% calories from FAT

Typical Restaurant Choice

6 oz. T-bone steak (with visible fat)
1 baked potato with butter and sour cream,
1/2 cup mixed vegetables,
1 slice apple pie,
12 oz. wine

1886 calories, 741 mg sodium (with no salt added)
14 gm fiber, 64% calories from FAT

So what does all this mean in nutrient terms?

Basically, this means the typical American diet is:

—too high in fat, protein, calories (sometimes), sodium, and cholesterol and too low in complex carbohydrates, fiber, and some vitamins and minerals.

You're thinking, "What a mess!" "I'm never going to remember all these things." Or "There're just too many things to change—so why don't I just forget about it."

Well, relax. It's not as complicated as it seems. All these nutrient problems are related and can be easily understood and solved. Allow me to explain.

For many of us, problems start with our choosing too many high fat foods and meals high in protein. (Meals high in animal protein usually tend to be high in fat, too.) And where there's fat, there's a whole bunch of calories. As an example of the problem, in 1991, Americans spent $3.9 billion buying fish and seafood in grocery stores, while they spent $26.7 billion on beef, pork, lamb, and veal. (Excess meat consumption also is helping to keep our saturated fat intake at an all-time high.)

If someone said to you, "Quick, think of some high-protein foods," you might imagine a thick, juicy, medium rare, 6-ounce steak—untrimmed of fat, of course, because as others will remind you, it's the best part. Did you also imagine it having 805 calories, 83 percent of which are from fat? Or maybe I'm catching you on a sunny Saturday morning and you're thinking of a two-egg omelette filled with 2 ounces of cheese, bubbling out of the side nearest you. Well, the omelette has 370 calories, 71 percent of which are from fat—not to mention the fried potatoes or sausage you could be picturing next to it!

And of course, when we eat typical American food, we add extra fat to our food one way or another—like oil in our frying pans, shortening in the mixing bowl, and butter or sour cream on the table.

So you see, an excess in animal protein (dairy foods, meats, eggs, etc.) can also lead to a high intake of cholesterol—and excess fat, in general. And in turn, this usually leads to excess calories.

So if we're making our portions of animal protein food smaller, eating less fatty foods, etc., what should we eat instead? The answer is complex carbohydrates. By eating foods such as fruits, vegetables, grains (rice, oats), whole-wheat bread, beans, legumes, and pasta, we can't help but increase the amount of fiber in our diets and improve the amount and combinations of vitamins and minerals, too.

If you haven't got it all down yet, don't panic. That's what the rest of this book is for.

I'm not suggesting you never drive through the golden arches again. I'm not even suggesting the frozen food section be roped off as a "restricted area—beware." And I'm not saying fast and frozen foods are BAD and home-cooked meals are GOOD, because there are better, healthier choices out there. . . yes, even in convenience land. We just need to know what they are.

Once we start pitching our dollars on the healthier choices, we're sending a vote to food companies and restaurants in favor of selling healthier products. So as time goes on, we may even have more healthful foods to choose from.

Nutrition is becoming a top priority for more and more people. But so is time and—as long as we all have taste buds and a desire to enjoy eating—taste.

The top three factors involved in choosing food should be:

• Nutrition

• Time

• Taste

If you're wondering why taste is rated third, hear me out. In order to really taste your food, you have to have time to enjoy eating it, which for some of us means taking less time to make it. And we won't have time or taste buds unless we are alive and well, which is where low-fat eating comes in—and thus the need for this book.

Why Use Percent Calories from Fat and What Does It Mean?

Before we go any further, there's something you should know. You may have already wondered, "Why is she using percent calories from fat and what does it mean anyway?" You should know there are two ways of judging whether something is low in fat. You can use grams of fat or the percent of calories from fat. The latter is a percentage based on the proportion of fat calories to total calories and therefore gives you a percentage. The first is an absolute amount based on the weight of fat in a particular product.

Currently, it's an on-going debate between the two. Some dietitians pledge allegiance to the grams-of-fat camp and others swear percent calories from fat is the best way to go. It really is a choice between the two because paying attention to both is terribly confusing and time consuming. The truth is, they both have weaknesses, but using grams of fat as a way of judging fat content has many more weaknesses, in my opinion. So basically this entire book is geared to using the percent of calories from fat criteria because it has fewer problems.

First of all, if the whole point is that you're trying to adhere to the "eat less than 30 percent of calories from fat" daily health guidelines, wouldn't you want to judge your meals by the same criteria? It makes sense that if most of your meals are less than 30 percent calories from fat, your overall intake is less than 30 percent calories from fat. That's the beauty of using percentages; they cross over boundaries. For example, if every item you put in your mouth during a meal is less than 30 percent calories from fat, then the whole meal will be less than 30 percent calories from fat. And if every meal during the day is less than 30 percent calories from fat, then your day's intake will be less than 30 percent calories from fat!

So because each meal is a separate entity, each one having less than 30 percent calories from fat, you can move on to the next meal without regard to the last. When using grams of fat, your daily allotment of fat grams has to be added up as the day goes on. For example, if you're supposed to eat 1,800 calories a day with less than 30 percent of those calories from fat, you need to have less than 60 grams of fat each day.

Here's how to calculate your fat calorie allowance. Say you eat 1800 calories a day. Multiply 1,800 calories by 30 percent. This tells you you can have 540 fat calories. Each gram of fat has 9 calories, so 540 fat calories divided by 9 gives 60 grams of fat.

Which brings me to another problem with using grams of fat. No one eats exactly the same amount of calories day in and day out. And no one has the time and energy to faithfully keep track of their grams of fat and total calories over a day's time. For example, if you eat 60 grams of fat, but for some reason your meals added up to only 1,400 calories that particular day, you will have eaten 39 percent of your calories from fat—hardly close to the less than 30 percent guidelines.

But, if for some reason you've already settled into the grams of fat groove, or if you're just plain curious, you can calculate grams of fat from the percent calories from fat information in this book by:

- Step 1:   Divide the percent calories from fat by 100.

- Step 2:   Multiply the calories per serving by this fraction.

- Step 3:   Take this new number and divide by 9 (the number of calories in 1 gram of fat).

Your answer tells you the grams of fat per serving.

And here's how to calculate percent of calories from fat from grams of fat.

- Step 1:   Take the grams of fat per serving and multiply by 9 (because there are 9 calories per gram of fat)

    _____grams of fat x 9 = _____ calories from fat

- Step 2:   Take the calories from fat and divide by the total calories per serving

    calories from fat

    _____ = _____ total calories

- Step 3:   Take this fraction and multiply by 100 to get the percentage of calories from fat

    _____ x 100 = _____ % calories from fat

Here's an example:

One serving of Orville Redenbacher's Smart Pop® popcorn contains 1 gram of fat. One multiplied by 9 equals 9 calories from fat. Nine divided by 50 total calories (per serving) equals 0.18. And 0.18 multiplied by 100 equals 18 percent of calories from fat.

Chapter

Focus on Fat:
Your Life Depends on It

People come up with all sorts of reasons for not caring that the way they eat may be hazardous to their health. "My father lived to be 90." "I've never been overweight." "You have to die of something." I've heard them all!

True, we do have to die of something, but the way we eat may strongly direct whether we die of *this* "something" at age 50 or 90. True, our genes partly determine our risk for these chronic diseases or possibly our response to the nutritional factors that relate to chronic disease. But for many of these diseases, we don't yet have a way of identifying who these susceptible people are.

Besides, who are we kidding? We're not just talking about one or two percent of Americans who happen to be born in a family dying primarily of chronic disease! Seventy percent of all deaths in the United States are related to cardiovascular diseases and cancer (numbers one and two in a distinguished list of chronic diseases).

In 1988, "low-fat eating" made the front page of most newspapers, thanks to the much appreciated report from the Surgeon General C. Everett Koop on Nutrition and Health. Dr. Koop positioned the diet on the front line of defense against chronic disease by saying, "If you are among the two out of three Americans who do not smoke or drink excessively, your choice of diet can influence your long-term health prospects more than any other action you might take."

Koop even confirmed that dietary fat is the number one bad guy, saying: "Of greatest concern is our excessive intake of dietary fat and its relationship to risk of chronic diseases such as coronary heart disease, some types of cancers, diabetes, high blood pressure, stroke, and obesity."

So, according to this government report, issued from America's consummate physician (so to speak), reducing our fat intake is the number one dietary priority of the nation. It's music to my ears. More specifically, the report said a high intake of total dietary fat is associated with increases in risk for obesity, some types of cancer, and possibly gallbladder disease. Furthermore, a high intake of saturated fats and, to a lesser degree, of dietary cholesterol is linked to increased risk of coronary heart disease.

Then, in 1989, the National Academy of Sciences released the 1,200-some-odd-page report entitled "Diet and Health—Implications for Reducing Chronic Disease Risk." And what do you know! The committee gave highest priority to the recommendation to reduce the total amount of fat in our diets. The report explained that it gave top billing to fat because "the scientific evidence concerning dietary fats and other lipids and human health is strongest and the likely impact on public health is greatest."

The report recommended Americans "reduce total fat to 30 percent or less of calories, reduce saturated fatty acid intake to less than 10 percent of calories, and reduce cholesterol to less than 300 milligrams daily." Well, that sure sounds like a lot of "reducing" needs to go on.

But fear not. There are certain foods we should eat more of. The report points out that most people should compensate for the loss of fat calories by eating greater amounts of complex carbohydrates (by choosing more vegetables, fruits, grains, cereals, and legumes).

The justification for the recommendations these two reports make rests on the role diet (particularly dietary fat) plays in five of the ten leading causes of death: Heart disease (number one), cancer (number two), stroke (number three), diabetes (number seven), and atherosclerosis (number ten). One statistic from the Surgeon General's report that really impressed me was that of the 2.1 million Americans who died in 1987, nearly 1.5 million (71 percent) were killed by diseases associated with poor diet. What are these alleged associations? Take a look at the chart that follows.

Changes in Diet that Can
Reduce the Risks of Certain Diseases

Disease	Eat Less Fat	Control Calories	Increase Starch & Fiber	Reduce Sodium	Control Alcohol
Heart Disease	X	X		X	
Cancer	X	X	X		X
Stroke	X	X		X	X
Diabetes	X	X	X		
Gastro-Intestinal Disease	X	X	X		X

An "X" indicates that making this change in the average American diet will reduce the risk for that disease. [Source: *Surgeon General's Report on Nutrition and Health, 1988.*]

After looking at the chart, it's plain to see how "eating less fat" became the most important dietary recommendation. There's a bonus in following this guideline, too. Eating less fat will also assist you in meeting the next recommendation—"control calories"—because "fat" has more than twice the calories per gram as carbohydrates and protein. High-fat foods, not surprisingly, tend to be high calorie foods.

Now, if you're ready, we'll move on to discuss each of America's top three health concerns individually—heart disease, obesity and dieting, and cancer. Then we'll finish the chapter by making sense of all the various diet guidelines that have come out within the past decade—from the American Heart Association to the National Cancer Institute.

Heart Disease

Can you say "No cholesterol?" I knew you could, because most people can and do—quite often in an average day. This is one nutrition term America has down pat.

Oddly enough, so do the food companies who plaster "No Cholesterol" on their packages of potato chips, bottles of vegetable oils, and cans of vegetable shortening. I hate to break the news to everyone, but these foods never had cholesterol! But, they've always been (and still are) high in fat.

Then again, there are those products, such as egg noodles, mayonnaise, eggs, or ice cream, that normally do contain cholesterol and now have no-cholesterol alternatives. Examples are "No Yolks" pasta or Mocha Mix, the second of which still comes in a high fat version. So now that you're totally confused, how can we tell the difference between cholesterol claims on products that never had cholesterol and products that really have been modified? And is this no cholesterol stuff as important as everyone thinks?

There are actually two meanings for the word "cholesterol." Dietary cholesterol is the amount of cholesterol in the food we eat, and serum cholesterol is the amount of cholesterol-containing lipids (fats) swirling through our bloodstreams.

High serum cholesterol (the main contributor to the bad publicity on cholesterol) is one of the three most important controllable heart disease risk factors. The other two are cigarette smoking and high blood pressure. Dietary cholesterol is just one of the many food constituents that help dictate our serum cholesterol levels. The others are high amounts of total fat, saturated fat, and excess calories. And out of all of these, total fat is the main boogie man.

Experts agree that one of the major determinants of high serum cholesterol levels in otherwise normal people is the total amount of fat eaten. Thus, the most powerful way to reduce our serum cholesterol levels is to reduce the total amount of fat we eat—especially saturated fat. Plus by lowering the total amount of fat in our meals (and lowering our percent of calories from fat), we will most likely also lower the amount of saturated fat, excess calories, and dietary cholesterol.

Still, it's a good idea to make a point of limiting the other constituents, namely cholesterol and saturated fat. And, as luck would have it, where there's cholesterol, there's saturated fat. Interestingly, it's not necessarily vice versa: Sometimes there is saturated fat in non-cholesterol foods, such as hydrogenated vegetable oils and coconut and palm oil, which are two naturally saturated vegetable oils.

You'll find cholesterol in all animal foods (meats, dairy products, fish, and poultry), but egg yolks and organ meats have much more than their fair share. Just remember where there's animal fat, there tends to be cholesterol. As the fat content goes down in a product containing cholesterol, so does the cholesterol content. A cup of whole milk, for example, has 35 milligrams of cholesterol and 51 percent of calories from fat, while nonfat milk has 5 milligrams of cholesterol and 5 percent of calories from fat.

It's true that we actually NEED cholesterol to form things like hormones and cell membranes in our bodies. But the human animal came prepared, and we actually produce this required cholesterol all by ourselves. So any cholesterol from the food we eat is extra.

What were our natural "no cholesterol" options before food companies created no-cholesterol eggs or mayonnaise? Vegetables, fruits, breads, cereals, grains, and legumes. But we tend to pour cheese or butter sauces over our pure and innocent vegetables, plop whipped cream on our fruits, spread gobs of cream cheese or butter on our bread (you get the picture), all of which add fat and cholesterol. Take white or whole-wheat flour. Knead it with butter and milk, and voila! You've got your basic croissant, with 60 milligrams of cholesterol each and around 50 percent of calories from fat!

What do we do about these other cholesterol-packed foods? First, keep in mind some are more packed than others. Obviously cholesterol-packed foods, such as egg yolks and organ meats, should be cut back when possible. But if you're going to reach into that egg carton, keep your hands off the full fat versions of sour cream, cheese, bacon, butter, and so on, and try to stretch out each yolk by sharing one with the one you love. Make scrambled eggs for two by mixing one egg with 1/2 cup egg substitute or three to four egg whites.

Second, remember the bottom line is the total amount of fat (percent calories from fat). You'll find some foods, such as certain shellfish, are low in total fat, but moderately high in cholesterol. Of what am I speaking? I'll save you the trouble and boredom of reading through your nearest food chart: The low-fat foods in the cholesterol hot seat are squid and shrimp.

In their defense, let me just add that, per ounce, these fishes have a much lower calorie and fat content than your average slice of beef or pork. The serving size is usually smaller (around 2 ounces) for these foods, too, compared with the three-egg omelette or the 6-ounce T-bone steak.

So, let's review. What most of us have actually heard, from scientific sources, about lowering our serum cholesterol levels applies to eating a low-fat diet. Certainly, eating less than 300 milligrams of cholesterol a day and limiting saturated fat is part of this low-fat way of eating. Just because something doesn't have cholesterol doesn't mean it's low in fat or good for you. Many of the chips, crackers, or non-dairy creamers, boasting "no cholesterol" have just as much fat as the regular rich items.

Serum Cholesterol Tests

Heart disease usually strikes without warning. (Only 20 percent of heart attacks are preceded by chest pains or angina.) And even though being thin is seen as an "end all" in our society, healthy arteries aren't necessarily part of the deal. Being thin doesn't automatically pardon you from having high blood pressure or high serum cholesterol.

And if you're young, congratulations are in order. You are at the BEST time in your life to start preventing heart disease! If you wait until you start feeling like a mere mortal, say around age 40, some damage has probably already occurred. It's best to get a running start in the race against heart disease. Recent evidence shows a possible two-year lag period from the time serum cholesterol levels are lowered and the time there is an actual reduction in the risk of heart disease.

I know preventing heart disease isn't the most thrilling challenge to have. But if high drama is what you want, I've got plenty of morbidity and mortality statistics I can show you. Will you settle for one? "Total serum cholesterol" levels greater than 200 mg/dl are considered "incompatible with optimal cardiovascular health." This person is at moderate to high risk for heart disease, depending on how much above 200 the serum cholesterol levels are. Here's the scary part: More than half of all middle-aged Americans have serum cholesterol levels greater than 200 mg/dl.

Taking "The Test"

Are you waiting until your 40th birthday to have your serum cholesterol measured? If you have a family history of heart disease—that is if relatives have died at an early age (before 50) of stroke or heart attack—some experts are now recommending that you be tested at age 20 and retested every three years. If you don't have heart disease in your family, first pat yourself on the back because you're rare. Then, take a cholesterol test when you're 30 and repeat the test every five years.

Now, for those of you hiding in your genes saying, "Either I'm born with it or I'm not," you should know that most of us are born with serum cholesterol levels of about 70 mg/dl. And between the ages of 1 and 17 our average serum cholesterol level is about 150. This is the level for three-fourths of the world's adult population—who don't tend to get heart disease.

Many of the heart attacks in America strike people with a serum cholesterol level between 200 and 250 mg/dl. Still, some people in that group don't have heart attacks. Why? We have no absolute answers, but my guess is that it has to do with our lifestyles. Smoking, using alcohol or drugs, high blood pressure, and not eating the right food all play a role. Dr. William Castelli, one of the leading national experts on the subject, says, "Start with your diet." I couldn't agree more.

Several different serum cholesterol tests are available, some more indicative (and expensive) than others. You've got your basic "total serum cholesterol" test at around $24, or you have your complete "lipid profile" (which measures low-density lipoprotein, high-density lipoprotein, total serum cholesterol, and other components) at approximately $30. You can usually be tested at any private hospital, or you can call your local American Heart Association for a referral.

Good and Bad Serum Cholesterol

All cholesterol is not created equal. Low-density lipoproteins (LDL) are light in weight or "low in density" because they're mostly fat. They're better known as "BAD" cholesterol because high levels of LDL in the blood usually mean high total serum cholesterol levels. These are associated with an increased risk of coronary heart disease because LDLs tend to deposit themselves on artery walls.

On the other hand, high-density lipoproteins (HDL) are heavy because they're mostly protein, and protein weighs more than water or fat. This provides more muscle to push bad cholesterol around and helps remove excess cholesterol from the artery wall. Higher levels of HDL in the blood are associated with lower rates of heart disease.

The most accurate way to measure your heart disease risk is by looking at the ratio of either total serum cholesterol to HDL or LDL to HDL. These two ratios continue to predict risk in people older than 55 years, unlike the straight total serum cholesterol measurement. Let's look at RISK:

Total Serum Cholesterol Measurement

Age	Moderate Risk	High Risk
2-19	>170	>185
20-29	>200	>220
30-39	>220	>240
>40	>240	>260

- Levels of 140 to 180 mg/dl are associated with the lowest rates of coronary heart disease.
- Levels of 180 to 200 mg/dl are associated with substantially lower heart disease incidence and favorable overall health status.
- At 250 mg/dl, you have twice the risk as at 200 mg/dl.
- At 300 mg/dl, your risk is four times higher than at 200 mg/dl.

Total Serum Cholesterol to HDL Ratio

- A ratio of 5.0 reflects high risk.
- 4.5 or higher is cause for concern (levels typical in affluent Western populations).
- At 3.5, risk is about half the standard (typical of levels found in countries with a low incidence of heart disease).

In general, pay attention to HDL levels of less than 40 mg.

LDL to HDL ratio in men 50 to 79 years of age:

- A ratio of 1.0 carries one half the average risk.
- At 3.6 the risk is considered average.
- A ratio of 6.3 carries two times the average risk.
- At 8.0, the risk is three times average.

Allow me to offer you some encouragement:

- Every 10 mg/dl increase in HDL cholesterol is associated with a 50 percent decrease in heart disease risk.
- It is estimated that for every 1 percent you lower your serum cholesterol, your risk for heart attack drops by 2 percent. More and more data show this is true for young or older alike.
- No environmental factor—smoking, exercise, stress reduction—has been shown to influence serum cholesterol and LDL-cholesterol more profoundly than DIET.

The Oat Bran Story

In the 1980s, oat bran sales skyrocketed. Ever wish you had stock in a particular product—after the fact? We definitely witnessed an oat bran boom. Newspapers and magazines constantly wrote about it. New food products featuring oat bran as an ingredient seemed to squeeze their way onto the supermarket shelves daily. So what's going on? What's the real story with oat bran? The answer is a simple two words: Soluble fiber.

Oats contain a type of fiber that is soluble in water. When eaten in recommended amounts, this fiber reduces serum cholesterol levels. The soluble plant fiber found in oats (called beta glucangum) appears to form a gel in the intestines and binds with bile acids. (Your body uses its stores of cholesterol to manufacture these digestive juices.) The undigestible fiber and the bile acids attached to it (carrying the cholesterol) pass right through the body. But this doesn't seem to be the only oat bran benefit.

Another mechanism in the intestines (involving the production of short-chain fatty acids) may also have value for lowering cholesterol. Unfortunately, we need more research to understand this, but it's in the works.

Sounds pretty straight forward, right? All you have to do is eat oat bran and your serum cholesterol will drop. Wrong! Here's the catch. All the studies showing health benefits with oats or oat bran were done as part of a low-cholesterol, low-fat diet. One researcher even estimated that about a third of the demonstrated reduction in serum cholesterol could be attributed to the oat bran factor. He attributed the rest to the infamous "Low-Fat Diet."

But don't get me wrong. Certainly all these studies are telling us something. Oats and oat bran, as particularly great sources of soluble fiber, can enhance the serum cholesterol lowering effects of a diet low in fat and cholesterol.

At a time when boxes of oat bran remain scarce and when mothers everywhere try to replace good old-fashioned oatmeal with oat bran hot cereal, I'm thrilled to pass on some truly liberating information. You don't have to eat "oat bran" cereal to acquire the benefits of the soluble fiber in oats. You can also eat plain old oats!

Because the bran part of the oat is particularly difficult to extract without collecting quite a bit of oat starch with it, there actually isn't a big difference between the amount of soluble fiber in oat bran versus regular oats. That's also why oat bran contains some calories. The recommended daily dose of oat bran is 2/3 cup (dry), which contributes 4 grams of water-soluble fiber. So for people out there who have been enjoying hot oatmeal for years, keep on enjoying it—without added butter or cream, of course!

What about all the oat bran diehards? Should they buy the finer or coarser (flakier) grinds? When first asked this question, my instinct was to answer "coarser." (I must confess that I do have a preference toward cooking with the coarser, flakier types.) Later it occurred to me that perhaps the finer, more granular types might blend with intestinal water and bile acids easier, therefore making itself more physiologically available and useful.

I frantically proceeded to fish around for some evidence one way or the other. My curiosity was captured. And the winner is . . . both! Currently, no specific information shows that one is better than the other. So my advice to you for now is to try them both and see which you like best.

Beyond Oat Bran

Oat bran has infiltrated supermarket shelves everywhere. From English muffins to frozen waffles, it's the star ingredient in many foods. You know you've made it when Mrs. Fields creates a cookie in your honor. (That's right! You can now buy oat bran cookies at Mrs. Fields.) What's next? Oat bran chips?

This may come as a shock to certain food companies, but oat bran does NOT have exclusive rights to "soluble fiber." Remember soluble fibers, as a group, are thought to help reduce the bad cholesterol, LDL, in the blood. It's just that oat bran and oatmeal have particularly impressive amounts of this type of fiber.

In fact, rice bran enthusiasts are eagerly trying to get their facts and figures together so they, too, can enter this profitable popularity contest.

Studies to determine the health benefits of rice bran continue. Some completed studies suggest blood cholesterol benefits; others suggest no significant reductions. In one recent study, rice bran was shown to be as effective as oat bran in lowering serum cholesterol levels.

I can tell you right now, packaging and selling rice bran will be a bit more tricky than oat bran. Of the 78 calories or so per ounce of rice bran, 40 percent is from fat. With oat bran, only 10 percent of calories is from fat. With such a significant amount of fat, mostly unsaturated, in rice bran, keeping the bran from turning rancid after a short time is a big challenge.

But before all of us start running around in search of the perfect bran, there is some more crucial information you should know. Many of the scientists conducting research on increasing the intake of water-soluble fiber suggested a VARIETY of food sources for the fiber. I'm afraid this is one of those boring but true cases where "variety" is the key. No quick-fix, fancy solution, just your run-of-the-mill "balanced and varied" diet.

Where then are some of these other potential sources of soluble fiber? We can pick up some in the produce section, and we can buy it in a can. Certain beans—kidney, white, and pinto—in amounts of about 1/2 cup (canned), come close to matching the power of oats. Let us not forget our friends the fruits and vegetables: 1/2 cup of broccoli, a small apple, 1/3 cup purple plums, a small orange, and 1/2 cup of carrots, all have a third to half the water-soluble fiber found in 1/3 cup of oat bran.

The lesson here is that we will probably never find the perfect bran since there are several different types of fiber. Each has specific physiological purposes and health benefits. Perfection, in this case, seems to come in the form of "variation."

Omega-3 Update

The Future for Fish Oils

It's been a while since Omega-3 fatty acids hit the press and airwaves as champions in the war against cholesterol build-up. (Sounds like a powerful bathroom cleanser, doesn't it?) Are these little fish oils going to swim out of the limelight as quickly as they swam in? I doubt it.

The Omega-3 fatty acids, which are polyunsaturated, by the way, apparently work by making it more difficult for blood to clot and by protecting blood vessel walls from cholesterol accumulation. For you and me, this means a reduced risk of artery blockage and heart attack. Fish oils somehow lower the levels of bad cholesterol and raise those for good cholesterol.

But it isn't as simple as it sounds. (Is it ever?) One study, in which people ate 7 ounces of fish every day, showed a decrease in serum triglycerides only. No change was seen in LDL or HDL levels.

And the fish oil supplement studies aren't any help either. Even to meet the lower end of the dose scale (4 grams of EPA a day) used in these studies would require popping 35 to 100 high-priced pills every day! And speaking of fish oil supplements, I have just a few more gripes. Supplement companies have chosen not to list the amount of cholesterol and the exact part of the fish's body the oil comes from on their product labels.

Does that matter? In my opinion, yes it does. A typical dose, as used in these studies, may add around 300 milligrams of cholesterol to your diet each day. If the fish oils are taken from the liver of the fish, they may contain pesticides or other contaminants. Because Omega-3 fatty acids are easily oxidized (meaning they link up with oxygen molecules) they will most likely increase our need for antioxidants, such as vitamin E or selenium. (Antioxidants will link up with oxygen instead of the Omega-3 fatty acids.) Work is still going on to test the various health attributes of the Omega-3s. But some studies suggest that a diet rich in fish oil can reduce levels of high blood fats. Omega-3s might also aid in keeping platelets in the blood from becoming less "sticky" and therefore less apt to form blood clots.

Along with their possible role in preventing coronary heart disease, Omega-3s are being studied for preventing breast cancer, high blood pressure, migraine headaches, and rheumatoid arthritis. Some studies suggest Omega-3s may reduce the number and size of some tumors, may increase the time elapsing before the appearance of tumors, and have the potential to serve as therapeutic agents for inflammatory diseases.

While the long-term effects of fish oil supplements are still unknown,we do know Omega-3s affect each person differently, and it's impossible to prescribe a specific dosage at this point. Fish oil supplements, according to a Food and Drug Administration (FDA) ruling, should be classified as "drugs," forcing companies to prove their safety and value. What does the FDA say to fish oil supplements continually being promoted as beneficial to health? They say, "There is no general recognition by qualified experts to warrant these marketing claims at this time."

The word from experts on the best way to get your Omega-3s is still "EAT FISH!" Can a recommendation be so generic about fish? It certainly can. All seafood contains Omega-3 fatty acids. The fattier fish just have more.

How much fish? Moderation is still the key. Most experts are recommending 2 to 4 servings of fish each week, or an average of nine ounces per week. Most Americans are still not measuring up. One source showed the average American has less than 20 ounces of fish a month—or less than five ounces a week. But that's nothing that a four-ounce serving of salmon or sardines can't cure.

There's no magical oil or potion. And no getting around it, folks. America has to aim toward a diet lower in total fat and saturated fat. It's probably best that we "Westerners" think of this fish oil business in terms of trying to replace some of our overflowing amounts of saturated fat with Omega-3 foods—seafood, beans, nuts, and nut oils. Has a study been done from this angle? Glad you asked. A 16-year study was done in Seattle, where fish was substituted for meat three times a week. The control groups had four times the incidence of fatal heart attacks as the fish eaters.

Typically, we need more and better research before we can remove all doubts that Omega-3s were solely (there's a nifty pun) responsible for these results. What is clear is that benefits from Omega-3s last only as long as they are consumed, and there's no evidence so far that pre-existing heart disease can be reversed by consuming these fatty acids.

Non-fish sources of Omega-3s are listed below, along with high Omega-3 and medium Omega-3 fish.

Non-Fish Omega-3 Foods

Food, edible portion, raw	Grams of linolenic acid per 100 mg.
Linseed oil	53.3
Rapeseed oil (canola)	11.1
Soybean oil	6.8
Walnut oil	10.4
Wheatgerm oil	6.9
Beans, common, dry	0.6
Soybeans, dry	1.6

Food, edible portion, raw	Grams of linolenic acid per 100 mg.
Beechnuts, dried	8.7
English walnuts	6.8
Leeks, freeze-dried, raw	0.7
Seaweed, spirolina, dried	0.8
Soybeans, green, raw	3.2
Soybeans, mature seeds, cooked	2.1

High Omega-3 Fish

(Providing 1 to 2 grams of Omega-3 fatty acids per 100 grams)

Salmon	Herring
Sable Fish	Fresh Tuna
Anchovies	Mackerel
Sardines	Lake Trout
Whitefish	

Medium Omega-3 Fish

(Providing 0.5 to 0.9 grams of Omega-3 fatty acids per 100 grams)

Halibut	Rockfish
Sea Trout	Bass
Oysters	Bluefish
Rainbow Trout	Ocean Perch
Pollock	

Controlling High Blood Pressure

It seems the time has come to add "SALT" to our list of four letter words. But isn't it true (you might debate) salt (also known as sodium chloride) is being cross-examined only because of its association with the mineral sodium? And shouldn't it really be SODIUM on trial?

Well, hear me out. One-third of the average American's sodium intake comes directly from the salt he or she dutifully adds at the table or when cooking. And the average American's sodium intake totals around 5,000 milligrams per day. So, if this average American took the salt shaker off the table—or better yet, stuck it way behind the baking powder in some hard-to-reach cupboard—couldn't we expect to drop to the 1,000 to 3,000 milligrams per day limits recommended by the American Heart Association and the National Academy of Sciences? The prosecution rests.

Why all this fuss over salt and sodium? In a word, HYPERTENSION. At least one of every four American adults have it—60 million people. About 95 percent of them are stuck with it for the rest of their lives because the cause is unknown. That's obviously the BAD news. The good news is there *are* several ways to help *control hypertension*.

Hypertension is a fancy name for high blood pressure. It's a major risk factor for the number one American killer, heart disease. It also is an underlying cause of America's number three cause of death, Stroke. It often develops without any symptoms when we reach age 30 or 40. And it's difficult to predict who will be that one person in four to get it! More bad news. But I can tell you right now, if your parents have it or had it, there's a good chance you will too! Here are a few more facts about hypertension.

- The incidence of severely high blood pressure is three times higher for blacks than for whites.
- The older you get, the higher your risk. (By age 74, half the U.S. population has hypertension.)
- If you're considered "obese," your risk is increased.
- If you're over 35, use oral contraceptives, and smoke, your risk is increased.
- If you have diabetes or kidney disease, your risk is high.

But no matter what, getting your blood pressure checked is the key. More than one-third of the 60 million people with hypertension don't even know they have it. And it's the high blood pressure that goes untreated that can lead to heart attack and stroke. If your blood pressure was normal the last time it was checked, be sure to get it rechecked every couple of years. And bring your kids with you. The National Heart, Lung, Blood Institute says, "High blood pressure in children represents a significant clinical problem."

High blood pressure treatment, other than medications, usually includes weight reduction if you're obese, limiting salt and sodium in your diet, controlling heavy drinking, and exercising. All of these are things we all should be doing for other reasons!

Some minerals, new on the hypertension scene, may help in the treatment and possibly the prevention of hypertension:

- *Magnesium:* Recent population studies suggest eating magnesium-packed foods, such as vegetables, fruits, whole grains, and low-fat dairy items, to ensure an adequate intake of magnesium.

- *Potassium*: The diet high in potassium may provide some protection in the arteries of people with high blood pressure. It may also lower blood pressure a little and protect the kidneys from related damage.

  Potassium is the mineral that made the banana the famous fruit it is. But potatoes, apricots, orange and grapefruit juice, and just about any kind of fruit and vegetable not cooked in water will add potassium to our diets. People with a history of kidney failure should check with their doctors before increasing their intake of these items.

  One researcher reported an increase of 10 millimoles of potassium in a retirement community—just one extra serving of fruit or vegetables—reduced the risk of stroke by 40 percent. Certainly, encouraging Americans to eat more fruits and vegetables is a good way to make sure we meet our Recommended Daily Allowance (RDA) for potassium.

- *Calcium:* Just when you thought it was safe to avoid dairy products, evidence turns up linking decreases in systolic blood pressure and higher intakes of calcium or calcium supplements. It seems to work best for people with previous intake of calcium well below the RDA who have high systolic blood pressure readings. (Systolic is the top number in the blood pressure reading.)

A small number of people with hypertension may even have a rise in blood pressure with calcium supplements. And, of course, we're not able to detect who these people are beforehand. At this point, though, experts only recommend we take in the RDA for calcium (800 mg per day, 1200 mg per day for ages 11 to 24 and pregnant women). Very little evidence supports a need for more than this amount.

The Case Against Sodium

The learned taste for salt will take about two months to be unlearned. As you eat less and less salt, your taste buds become more aware of the salt and sodium that's there. You might ask, "Aren't only certain people sensitive to salt?" (This refers to the people whose blood pressure rises from excessive sodium in their diet.)

Well, yes, but let me explain. We need to be concerned about two "salt-sensitive" groups: those who already have high blood pressure and those who don't (yet). It has been estimated that 30 to 60 percent of people with essential hypertension (high blood pressure not caused by medications or other illnesses) can expect a significant drop in blood pressure (5 to 8 points) in response to salt restriction. Sometimes, after about 7 months of a mild sodium-restricted diet, people can reduce or completely eliminate their blood pressure medication, which, by the way, can have many side effects.

Obviously, if you add up the numbers (30 to 60 percent of a hypertensive group of possibly 15 percent of the total population, plus 25 percent in the remaining nonhypertensive category), it's far from 100 percent. Ah! There's the rub. Why then should everyone go out of their way to limit the criminal mineral, sodium?

If reduced sodium will help protect even 20 percent of our population against potential stroke, heart attack, and kidney failure . . . and if we can still "taste saltiness" at these learned lower levels of salt and sodium . . . and as long as it is a reasonable reduction using basic steps, like no salting food at the table and limiting heavily salted processed foods, and not a severe restriction. . . the question isn't WHY, but WHY NOT?

Take soy sauce, or as I call it, "sodium sauce." You can buy the reduced-sodium soy sauce, cutting sodium in half without sacrificing flavor. At least I don't notice a difference, although I'm not really an expert on soy sauce.

Here are some sodium aliases, besides salt:

- seasoning salts (garlic salt, onion salt, etc.)
- MSG (monosodium glutamate)
- soy sauce
- brine (salt and water)
- broth and bouillon
- sodium compounds, including: sodium phosphate, sodium benzoate, sodium bicarbonate (baking soda), sodium hydroxide, sodium propionate, sodium sulfite, and baking powder
- AND any other compounds with the word "sodium" in them. (There are more than 70!)

Check the amount of sodium listed per serving on the label to truly know the combined effect of the sodium-containing ingredients.

If you tend to shake your salt . . .
take the Salt Shaker Test

1. Cover a plate with wax paper or foil.
2. Salt the make-believe plate of food as you would normally.
3. Measure the salt into the appropriate size teaspoon:

> 1/8 teaspoon of salt = 250 mg of sodium
>
> 1/4 teaspoon of salt = 500 mg of sodium
>
> 1/2 teaspoon of salt = 1,000 mg of sodium
>
> 1 teaspoon of salt = 2,000 mg of sodium

Now, multiply this amount by the number of times you grab the salt shaker in a day.

Obesity and Dieting

Like clockwork, the first few months in the new year and then the summer season simultaneously bring with them irritating commercials for countless weight-loss programs. The profit-driven diet programs aren't dumb; they're capitalizing on the surge of good intentions and newly sworn goals (not to mention the fear of swimsuits) that typically accompany this time of year.

Americans can't seem to shake their attachment to two modern dieting criteria: We want whatever we do to be quick and painless. We know it—and the weight-loss program people know it. The difference is they stand to make a profit every year because of it. And all we get is more frustrated, sometimes a bit heavier than we were, and, of course, we get a bill.

The bottom line is, these low-calorie diets just don't take the fat off for good. Here's why:

#1.   These diets are designed for quick "weight" loss, while losing body fat, which is what we really want, has to happen SLOWLY. In other words, if you're losing the pounds quickly, you can bet it isn't FAT you're losing. It could be body water, the breakdown of muscle tissue or essential carbohydrate stores. Keep in mind that in the best of circumstances you can only lose about two pounds of FAT a week; for some of us it might only be one pound a week.

#2.   Many of these diets are too low in calories. Your brain alone requires 150 grams of glucose energy per day. Your body prefers to get its glucose energy from carbohydrates, or, if it has to, from protein stores, also called lean body mass. So, just to preserve our musculature and keep our brain happy and productive, we need AT LEAST 600 calories in the form of mostly carbohydrates with about 1 gram of protein per kilogram of body weight (about 275 calories from protein for someone who weighs 150 pounds). But don't run off yet to check the calories on your diet shake. You also need some fat calories to balance your meals and contribute necessary fat-soluble vitamins, etc.

Which all means that most of us should never go on a diet that feeds us less than 1,000 calories a day. Not only is it counterproductive to losing the excess body fat that we're so anxious to lose (when we eat less than this our body starts conserving energy and actually burns and needs fewer calories than if we ate a little more), but we're risking our medical and nutritional safety as well.

#3.   The whole philosophy of "dieting" works against long-term loss of body fat. These diets are programs that we learn to suffer through for a short period of time, when what obviously needs to happen is long-term life changes if we want the loss of body fat to also be for a lifetime. I know this isn't going to be a popular statement but someone has to say it. It's our lifestyle—the way we usually eat and exercise—that got us into this dieting dilemma. Eventually returning to the same high-fat, high-calorie, sedentary lifestyle isn't going to break the cycle permanently.

#4.   Our suspicions should be raised by the very fact that most of these diet programs encourage you to depend on their particular products. Some even package their own salad dressings and vitamin supplements.

So how DO we lose weight safely and surely? First of all, we need to shift our focus from a "loss of pounds" to a "loss of body FAT." If scales were never invented, we would only have the way we feel and our appearance from which to judge, and isn't this what we should really be concerned about?

And you can encourage your body to use its extra fat by doing two things:

But I must warn you neither of these is easy or quick. They both involve pretty major changes in the way you've been doing business. And these changes should be permanent in order to keep your fat loss off for good.

#1.   Start eating a low-fat diet.

#2.   Make aerobic exercise a regular part of your life.

Rationale for Change

It has always made sense to me that fat from food would be more likely than carbohydrates to be deposited as fat in our bodies because the human body prefers to fuel itself with carbohydrate calories. Well, now I have some proof. It involves the Thermic Effect of Food (the "energy expended," or the caloric cost, of digestion, absorption, and storage of calories from fat, protein, and carbohydrate).

The body seems to handle the fat calories we eat more efficiently than equal calories from carbohydrates. This means it burns fewer calories taking care of the fat we just ingested than the carbohydrates. This is bad for us because we want the body to use as many calories as possible so we won't have unspent calories (so to speak) that will need to be "stored" as body fat. Don't underestimate how this might influence your weight control. The thermic effect of food accounts for approximately 10 percent of the calories we burn in a day.

Let's talk a bit more about why our bodies prefer to use carbohydrates as the main fuel and dietary fat for storage (energy for a rainy day). Well, for one thing, it costs the body too much energy to convert dietary carbohydrate to stored fat. One researcher recently calculated the storage of fat from dietary fat (with a caloric cost of 7 percent) is greatly favored over the energy-intensive carbohydrate-to-fat conversion (costing 28 percent).

Putting it into simpler terms, research has shown that adults gain weight much easier on a high-fat diet than on a diet consisting mostly of carbohydrate. Chalk one more up to the low-fat way of eating!

For many people, the fat loss process may be complicated by an internal control system—commonly referred to as the "set-point theory"—or a strong genetic influence that helps determine our basal metabolic rate (the amount of calories needed to sustain our bodies in a resting state) and how much fat each person carries and where. There are only two key lifestyle elements found to lower the theoretical "set point." Guess which two? Regular exercise and a low-fat diet.

I admit extremely overweight people may need some encouraging weight loss before they can collect the courage to face up to more effective and permanent lifestyle changes. Changing the way we eat and exercise requires extra personal motivation and external support. And that's where some of these commercial diet programs can help. The trick is finding a program that helps you with the behavioral aspects of your weight problem, teaches you the basics of eating a LOW-FAT diet, rich in essential nutrients for a lifetime, and includes an exercise component. They should also encourage you never to eat less than 1,200 calories a day.

Cancer and Diet

America is obsessed with cancer. Even Hollywood uses this disease to reach out to our emotions. Take, for example, the Academy-Award-winning film, "Terms of Endearment." I don't know about you, but I cried through the entire second half of this film.

But there is some news about cancer—and it happens to be good news. One-third of the cancer deaths in this country can be prevented through changes in our diet. If that hasn't impressed you, maybe this will. If America took to heart (and mouth) the dietary recommendations to prevent cancer—eating a diet low in fat, high in fiber with plenty of fruits and vegetables—200,000 lives would be saved each year!

How can we save those lives? Let's start by looking at two ways to prevent cancer through diet:

- Make sure you have plenty of the "good guys." (These are nutrients that help protect body cells from the "bad guys" or potential carcinogens.)
- Make sure you minimize your contact with the "bad guys." (These are substances that have a negative influence on your body's cells.)

Undoubtedly there are some people with their shoulders shrugging or arms waving who are declaring that "everything causes cancer!" So, why bother?

Why not utilize the nutrients that help protect your body cells from the dangers of carcinogens? I think this is a winning strategy in the battle against cancer. Of course, if you're going out of your way to build up your body's defenses against carcinogens, then it also makes sense to avoid close contact with the very enemies you're guarding yourself against.

So, okay, enough with the pep talk.

The Bad Guys

First, a rundown on some substances that are talked about in the media today. (At this point, however, no evidence is thought to exist proving these substances individually make a major contribution to cancer risk in the U.S.)

Nitrites: Sodium nitrite (and sometimes sodium nitrate) is a well-known additive used mainly to "pinken" and preserve processed meats, such as hot dogs, ham, bologna, salami, sausage, corned beef, bacon, and cured fish. Nitrites can convert into carcinogenic nitrosamines. More nitrosamines can form from very hot charbroiling, barbecuing, and frying—or in leftovers. So try to stay away from these on a daily basis.

Alfatoxins: These are formed by a certain type of mold that tends to grow on peanuts, corn, and cottonseed crops. Airtight packaging and refrigeration help protect nuts and corn kernels from forming molds. Salt added to nut butter also will help. If you don't do anything else, be sure to throw out any moldy or abnormal-looking nuts or corn kernels.

Natural carcinogens: Mother nature creates carcinogenic substances, too. They're found in produce such as mushrooms, potatoes, and rhubarb. But it isn't necessary, I repeat, is not necessary, to stop eating these vegetables. Just inspect them closely for bad spots and sprouts. Cut them out to about an inch on all sides. And, don't eat the spoiled ones. (Although you probably weren't going to do that anyway.)

Now on to the biggest bad guy of them all—FAT.

In epidemiological (meaning the comparison of population groups) and animal studies, a high-fat diet was indeed associated with a higher risk of certain cancers (mainly colon, breast, and prostate cancers). Or looking at it in a more positive way, switching to a low-fat diet will likely decrease the risk of these cancers.

Some researchers might argue that the question of whether the amount of fat in our diet is related to certain cancers is, at this point, still considered a toss-up. But whenever anything is being "tossed up," I always say, "Better safe than sorry." You better duck or be pretty well prepared to catch it!

There ARE indeed many studies that have suggested that a high-fat diet (no matter what type of fat) does increase your risk of these cancers. But whenever you study the effects of a diet high in fat, you're usually also—whether you want to or not—studying a diet high in total calories and protein. So far it's been difficult to completely separate these factors and note their individual effects.

The Good Guys

I'll get right to the point. Diets high in plant foods (fruits, vegetables, legumes, and whole-grain cereals), as part of a low-fat diet, are associated with a decrease in cancer of the lung, colon, esophagus, and stomach. There are several specific nutrients thought to be related to this protective effect.

Fiber

Fiber is thought to dilute potential cancer-forming substances by adding bulk that cannot be absorbed by the body. In addition, fiber decreases the time our intestinal wall is exposed to dangerous substances by escorting them quickly southward—if you know what I mean. It's suspected that the particularly insoluble fiber found in most whole grains and vegetables may protect the body against colon cancer. Other possible ways fiber protects the colon have also been proposed. Among them are: neutralizing various toxic metabolites by lowering the pH of the colonic lumen and binding with potential toxicants, which are then removed as waste along with the fiber.

Given there is still much to know and more research to be conducted about the different types of fiber (insoluble and soluble) and how one or more may aid in cancer prevention, experts recommend consuming a variety of fiber-containing foods.

What if I told you there was this great new high-fiber supplement you could inexpensively take several times a day that could increase your daily fiber total by 10 grams? Would you be willing to try it out? Would it help if I added that this is half the amount of fiber recommended by the National Cancer Institute (20 to 30 grams of fiber a day)?

What if I told you it wasn't a supplement at all, but a common food we can easily buy in our supermarkets or order in restaurants? Shouldn't you be even more interested in this high-fiber food? What I'm asking you to do is take a fresh look at plain old fruits and vegetables.

Actually, there are quite a few different fruits and vegetables that give us as much fiber as a health food "fiber bar" or a small scoop of bran. All fruits and vegetables, of course, contain some fiber and contribute to the "recommended daily amount" of 20 to 30 grams.

Let's admit one thing. Most of us don't sit down at the end of the day and add up how many grams of fiber we ate from whole grains and fruits and vegetables.

What would we do if our grand total was shy a few grams anyway? (Maybe swallow down another scoop of bran?)

Keep reading for more information on fruits and vegetables and the actual number of servings recommended for the best health.

Antioxidants

Most of us already know about the fiber connection. Cereal companies made sure of that. But which are the other body protectors? In a word, produce.

Just as knights were in danger without their metal armor, so a cell membrane should never leave home without an antioxidant. These protectors block attacks, reducing or neutralizing the effects of cancer-forming chemicals. Where can we buy these coats of armor? Beta carotene (and vitamin A), vitamins C and E, and the mineral selenium are your potential antioxidants.

Beta carotene is thought to be particularly effective at protecting against squamous-cell carcinoma (a common type of lung cancer). One study showed people with low levels of serum beta carotene were at least four times as likely to develop lung cancer as others.

How much is enough? The National Cancer Institute diet recommendations translate roughly into about 6 milligrams of beta carotene a day (about half a carrot). The typical American nibbles on only 1.5 milligrams a day. Popeye was on to something because spinach ranks number one in the top five beta carotene-rich foods, followed by carrots, broccoli, cantaloupe, and sweet potatoes. Not that I have anything against apples, but perhaps the saying should have been "a carrot a day . . ." Most of these foods also happen to be pretty good vitamin C providers, along with citrus fruits, of course. Vitamin C is the other antioxidant (when consumed in food) with some prospects of helping protect the body against some types of cancer.

Any Questions?

In the U.S. Surgeon General's report on Nutrition and Health released in 1987, fruits and vegetables as a group were listed as being associated with the prevention of lung, breast, colon, prostate, bladder, and stomach cancer. Specifically, fiber was listed as a fighter of breast and colon cancer.

Shortly after that, the National Academy of Sciences report on diet and health stressed that eating at least five servings of fruits and vegetables was an important disease preventing part of the highly recommended low-fat diet. A "serving" is 1/2 cup or 1 whole fruit (unless it's an exceptionally large fruit), or 6 ounces (3/4 cup) of pure fruit juice, or 1/4 cup of dried fruit.

In terms of the possible cancer prevention attributes of produce (fiber, vitamins A and C) some choices are better than others. The following lists are based on 1/2 cup servings or 1 whole fruit, unless otherwise noted.

Vitamin A rich fruits and vegetables

(These selections supply at least 50 percent of the RDA for vitamin A.)

Cantaloupe	Bok choy
Carrots	Apricots (3 whole)
Greens	Winter squash
Sweet potatoes	Spinach (1/2 cup cooked or 1 cup raw)

(These selections supply at least 25 percent of the RDA for vitamin A.)

Nectarines	Papayas
Broccoli	Tomatoes
Romaine lettuce (1 cup fresh)	
Loose leaf lettuce (1 cup fresh)	

Vitamin C rich fruits and vegetables

(These selections supply at least 50 percent of the RDA for vitamin C.)

Grapefruit (half)	Kiwi fruit
Oranges	Cantaloupe
Papaya	Strawberries
Orange juice	Broccoli
Brussels sprouts	Cauliflower
Green peppers	Green peas

(These selections supply at least 25 percent of the RDA for vitamin C.)

Grapes (1 cup)	Honeydew
Raspberries	Grapefruit juice
Tomato juice	Asparagus
Bok choy	Cabbage
Greens	Potatoes
Tomatoes	Spinach, (1/2 cup cooked, 1 cup raw)

Fruits with 3 grams or more of fiber per serving:

1/2 cup raspberries	1 apple
1 grapefruit	1 orange
1 pear	2 dried figs
4 prunes	

Vegetables with 3 grams or more of fiber per serving:

1 potato	1/2 cup corn
1/2 cup Brussels sprouts	1/2 cup eggplant, cooked
1/2 cup peas	1/2 cup winter squash, mashed

*What about bananas or strawberries? Or carrots, broccoli, spinach and cauliflower? They'll give you at least 2 grams of fiber, so don't leave them off your list.

What are Crucifers?

These are from the cabbage family. Indoles, chemical substances found in these vegetables, also enhance the body's cancer defense system. The American Cancer Society recommends we eat several servings a week. Some of the most common cruciferous vegetables are broccoli, cabbage, cauliflower, Brussels sprouts, kale, and turnips.

What it boils down to is basic good healthy eating. Boring but true. If we could just get Americans to eat more fruits, vegetables, and whole grains—as part of a low-fat diet. Ah! Wouldn't it be nice?

Diet Guidelines to Live By

It seems we have guidelines for almost everything—from safe sex to preventing disease through diet. Of course, I'm only going to talk about the latter.

Perhaps you haven't noticed, but the various leading health agencies and officials have spent the last few years coming up with their own packaged diet guidelines for the American public—some for preventing only heart disease, others for preventing some cancers, and still others for general good health.

THE LEADING DIETARY GUIDELINES

Title of document and organization	Total Fat	Saturated fat	Polyun- saturated fat	Cholesterol
Dietary Goals For the United States, 2nd ed. U.S. Senate Select Committee on Nutrition and Human Needs, 1977	Reduce to 27-33% of total calories	Reduce to 8-12% of total calories	Intake should be 8-12% of total calories	Reduce to 250-350 mg per day
Dietary Guidelines for Healthy American Adults. American Heart Assoc.–Nutrition Committee, 1986	Less than 30% of total calories	Less than 10% of total calories	Less than 10% of total calories	Reduce to 100 mg per 1000 calories, not to exceed 300mg/day
Recommended Dietary Allowances, Committee on Dietary Allowances, Food and Nutrition Board, National Research Council, National Academy of Sciences, 1980	Reduce to no more than 35% of total calories		Reduce to 10% of total calories	No more than 300 mg per day
Cholesterol Consensus Conference, National Institutes of Health, 1984	Less than 30% of calories			250-300 mg per day
Year 2000 Dietary Objectives of NCI, National Cancer Institute, 1986	Less than 30% of total calories			
National Cholesterol Education Program Adult Treatment Panel Report, 1987 Step 1 of Dietary Treatment:	Should be less than 30% of calories	Should be less than 10% of calories		Should be less than 300 mg per day
Step 2 of Dietary Treatment:	Should be less than 30% of calories	Intake should be less than 7% of calories	Should be less than 200 mg per day	
U.S. Surgeon General's Report "Nutrition and Health," 1988	Reduce consumption of fat (especially saturated fat) and cholesterol			
National Academy of Sciences "Diet and Health—Implications for Reducing Chronic Disease Risk,"1989	Reduce total fat to 30% or less of calories	Reduce to less than 10% of calories		Reduce to less than 300 mg per day
National Cancer Institute, 1992, promotes 5-a-day fruit and vegetable campaign				

Complex Carbohydrates	Fiber	Sugar	Sodium	Calcium
Increase complex carbohydrates and naturally occurring sugar to 45-51% of total calories	Increase	Reduce to 8-12% of total calories		
Increase to 50-55% or more of total calories with emphasis on increased complex carbohydrates			Reduce to 1 gram per 1000 calories not to exceed 3 grams	
		Reduce intake	Safe and adequate range of sodium is about 1100 -3300 mg/day	800 mg the Recommended Daily Allowance
Several servings daily of : • vit. A rich fruits and vegetables • vit. C rich fruits and vegetables Several servings weekly of: • crucigerous vegetables	Increase to 20-30 grams per day			
Increase consumption of whole grain foods and cereals, vegetables (including beans and peas), and fruits		Those vulnerable to dental cavities should limit use of sugar	Reduce intake of sodium	Adolescent girls and women should increase calcium intake
Eat greater amounts of complex carbohydrates			Limit daily salt to 6 grams or less	Maintain adequate calcium intake
Eat at least 5 servings of fruits and vegetables every day				

This surge in diet guidelines is rather bittersweet for me. While I'm thrilled they're finally paying tribute to the relationship between diet and disease, there now seem to be too many guidelines for the health-conscious consumer to sort through. There are just too many diet guidelines telling us to do too many different things pertaining to too many diseases.

So I decided to end this guideline quandary here and now by organizing the assorted guidelines in a table. I then selected the most rigid or specific guideline for each nutrient (better safe than sorry) and . . . ta da! A new set of guidelines, the "bottom line" guidelines were born, with only one rule to follow for fat, one for cholesterol, sodium, etc. These are the guidelines that are considered in the remainder of the book as far as recipes, restaurant suggestions, etc.

Bottom Line Guides:

- Reduce total fat to 30 percent or less of calories.
- Reduce saturated fat to less than 10 percent of calories
- Reduce polyunsaturated fat to less than 10 percent of calories
- Reduce dietary cholesterol to 250 to 300 mg per day
- Increase carbohydrates to 50 to 55 percent or more of total calories with emphasis on increased complex carbohydrates (fruits, vegetables, starches, grain products, beans)
- Eat at least five servings of fruits and vegetables every day

And for specific fruit and vegetable guidelines:

- Several servings daily of
  - vitamin A rich fruits and vegetable
  - vitamin C rich fruits and vegetables
- Several servings weekly of cruciferous vegetables
- Increase fiber to 20 to 30 grams per day
- Reduce sugar (refined carbohydrate) to 8 to 12 percent of total calories
- Limit sodium to the safe and adequate range of about 1,100 to 3,300 mg per day
- Maintain adequate calcium intake. The recommended daily allowance is 800 mg (1,200 mg for ages 11 to 24 and pregnant women)

But the greatest of all these is FAT. Always remember the guideline to eat a diet low in fat is the common denominator between the diet recommendations to prevent heart disease, obesity, and those for cancer and the link to all other diet recommendations (except possibly sodium and calcium).

For example, if someone is eating a diet low in fat (less than 30% of calories from fat) they are most likely also eating a diet low in saturated fat and cholesterol, since saturated fat and cholesterol are usually found together in fatty foods.

And the reduction in fat is considered much more significant for the American public in the prevention of disease than the others, such as reducing sugar and sodium. For example, the only disease that excessive sugar in the diet directly causes is dental caries! So please keep all this in perspective. I thought it was vital you be given all the guidelines so you could finally see them all together and how they really fit. For instance, there are at least seven different guidelines out for fat, but they are all pretty much saying the same thing. Eat less than 30 percent of calories from fat.

When fat is being reduced in the diet, some type of food will need to be increased. What's the missing piece to this puzzle? This is where the guidelines for increasing complex carbohydrates, fruits, and vegetables, and fiber fits in to complete the whole low-fat eating picture.

Then along came the long-awaited Food Pyramid in 1992, which graphically showed Americans which food groups should compose most of our diet (breads and cereals group and the fruit and vegetable groups) and which food groups should compose less (dairy and the meat and protein group).

The position of distinction (at the bottom of the pyramid) was awarded to the bread and cereal group, because it is suggested we eat at least 6 servings a day. The next section of the pyramid is shared by the fruit and vegetable groups, given the recommendation to eat at least 2 to 3 servings of each per day. Near the top of the pyramid, you'll find the dairy and meat groups because it is suggested we eat no more than 2 to 3 servings of each per day.

At the very top of the pyramid we find the fats and sugars groups. Much to my daughter's chagrin, this group wasn't given any recommended servings, but was just given a "limited" label.

What we all need to remember is that there are still low and high fat choices within each of these general groupings. Even in the bread and cereal group, there are high-fat bread and cereal choices (high-fat granola, croissants, muffins, etc.). And in the meat and dairy groups there are low-fat and fat-free choices (skinless chicken breast, low-fat fish, nonfat sour cream, yogurt, or cottage cheese, and so on).

Food Guide Pyramid

A Guide to Daily Food Choices

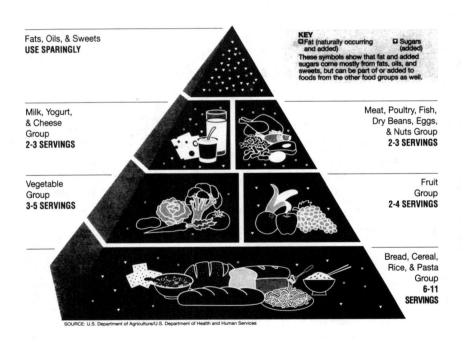

SOURCE: U.S. Department of Agriculture/U.S. Department of Health and Human Services

Use the Food Guide Pyramid to help you eat better every day. . .the Dietary Guidelines way. Start with plenty of Breads, Cereals, Rice, and Pasta; Vegetables; and Fruits. Add two to three servings from the Milk group and two to three servings from the Meat group.

Each of these food groups provides some, but not all, of the nutrients you need. No one food group is more important than another — for good health you need them all. Go easy on fats, oils, and sweets, the foods in the small tip of the Pyramid.

More Words on Exercise

There is an unspoken decree among some exercise and nutrition professionals to say a few qualifying words about the importance of exercise when good nutrition is being discussed, and vice versa. Well, the time has come for this nutritionist to progress beyond her simplified declaration that "aerobic exercise also is an essential part of a healthful (disease-preventing) lifestyle."

Far from what movies such as "Pumping Iron" or "Perfect" might lead you to believe, there IS more to exercise than flashing your favorite muscle groups, "toning," or feeling "the burn." In fact, there are so many wonderful health benefits to exercise (other than feeling more invigorated), that I can ask you confidently, "How many really good reasons do you need to start exercising regularly and aerobically for your health?" What? Three at least? All right, I'll name four, but you drive a hard bargain.

But first, let me mention that the operative concept here is "AEROBIC exercise," which is a fancy way of saying exercise that requires oxygen. Aerobic exercise is characterized by unfluctuating type exercise with consistent breathing, such as running, bicycling, swimming, walking fast, etc., and not so much stop and start as in baseball or tennis. So, in order to prevent visions of leotards jumping up and down from interfering with your reading enjoyment, from here until the end of this chapter, when I write "exercise" I'm referring to "aerobic exercise."

Reason #1: Increasing "Good Blood Cholesterol"

We've all heard about "bad cholesterol" and what we can do to help lower it. Well, here's blood cholesterol's better half—HDL (high-density lipoprotein) or "good cholesterol."

Increased levels of HDL in the blood have been associated with a decrease in the risk of coronary heart disease.

There are only a couple of things that have been shown to increase our circulating HDLs, besides certain medications. These are body fat loss in overweight people and aerobic exercise. Studies have shown that exercise and weight loss (in the overweight) together will increase HDLs the most.

Reason #2: Loss of Body Fat (Weight Loss)

Some people would rather take their chances on the latest "diet" than exercise regularly. But weight loss is such a common result of exercise that it is almost impossible for people in research studies involving regular exercise NOT to lose weight in a big way.

When you compare lost pound to lost pound, exercise has a more powerful effect on increasing HDLs than "dieting" alone. And body fat lost through exercise is more likely to stay off, too! But here's the catch. It usually takes a little longer to lose a pound through exercise.

There are no definite answers as to why all these wonderful things occur as a result of exercise, but I can tell you that a certain enzyme called lipoprotein lipase (an enzyme involved in forming and converting lipoproteins, the fat carriers in the blood) is being carefully watched by researchers. They have already discovered that exercise causes a greater change in levels of this enzyme than does dieting alone.

Reason #3: Decreased Triglyceride Levels

High triglycerides (one type of fat particle circulating in the blood) are currently thought to be a risk factor for heart disease when serum cholesterol levels are also high. According to some studies, exercise may encourage a decrease in blood triglycerides (after a meal) by removing triglyceride-rich fatty particles from the blood faster and possibly helping to reduce the risk of heart disease.

Reason #4: Decreased Blood Pressure

In research where people start on regular exercise programs there seems to be a significant decrease in their blood pressure that could be advantageous if blood pressure started off on the high side. But again, it's difficult to ascertain whether this is a consequence of the exercise or the loss in body fat that usually results from the exercise.

So there are four great reasons to think twice about enhancing your new low-fat way of eating by making exercise a regular (and enjoyable) part of your life!

Chapter 3

Shopping Savvy

Every time you step into a supermarket, thousands of products confront you, hundreds of exhausting buying decisions await you. Misleading packaging ads accost you at every corner. The supermarket—why it's a jungle in there!

The answer is shopping savvy. Years ago, the simple wisdom was "Shop the perimeter of the store and you'll avoid all the bad foods." That's unfortunately not possible. We've got to penetrate the dreaded "center" of the store—unless we are willing to exist without vitals such as flour, cereal, and even toilet paper. (I thought you would see it my way.)

Next, we must become "food label literate." This also involves developing a keen critical eye through which we view food advertisements so we aren't so easy to impress. You'll see what I mean when we go over some examples of deceptive advertising.

Label Literacy

Food companies use all sorts of alluring nutrition terms to help sell their products. These terms often deceive shoppers by suggesting a product is more healthy than it actually is.

Exhibit A

Take your average potato chip. The potato chip has always been and always will be a high-fat, high-sodium snack. Because vegetable oils and shortening are typically used to make them, they happen to NOT CONTAIN CHOLESTEROL.

So what, pray tell, do you see plastered across some potato chip bags? "No Cholesterol" of course. In isolation, this is a good thing, but it certainly doesn't cancel out the fact that the chip oozes with fat and sodium. (The "No Cholesterol" banner also advertises vegetable oils and shortenings—as if they ever had cholesterol!)

Exhibit B

"All Natural" or "100 Percent Natural" doesn't mean a whole lot in dietary guideline terms. After all, lard, salt, sugar, and butter are all perfectly "natural," but that doesn't mean you should sit down to a big bowl of sugary fat!

Then there's the "95 Percent Fat-Free" advertising claim you'll find on everything from turkey bologna to ice cream. Food advertisers are definitely faithfully following the "if you can't say anything nice" rule here. Because they could label it the other way—as 5 percent fat by weight. Don't let this fool you, though. This doesn't tell you anything about its PERCENT OF CALORIES FROM FAT, which is a more accurate way of judging fat content.

Many of the processed meats awarded this "95 Percent Fat-Free" status have, in fact, over half of their calories from fat! How can this be? When in doubt, check out the label. In most cases, you'll find the second ingredient is something that carries weight without calories (such as water), helping fat out in terms of its weight percentage but not the percentage that really counts—the percent of calories from fat.

Label Literacy Lesson #1

In May of 1994, a new food label appeared on packaged food items as mandated by law.

Currently nutrition information is voluntary for many raw foods such as fresh fruits and vegetables, raw meat, fish, and poultry. The new food label includes a good deal of information not included on the old label, such as saturated fat, sugars, fiber, cholesterol, and total calories from fat. Here's a summary of the changes:

- *Standardized serving sizes:* Previously, if a product was high in fat, a company could make a serving size smaller to "reduce" its fat content. Now all serving sizes will be standardized based on food consumption surveys.

- *Saturated fat:* This type of fat, when consumed excessively, is particularly likely to lead to clogged arteries, which often leads to heart disease. The government says that Americans should consume no more than 30 percent of calories from fat; saturated fat should supply no more than 10 percent of the total fat intake.

  Food labels will have to indicate total fat grams, as well as grams of saturated fat, but the percent of calories derived from fat is still not mandatory.

- *Dietary fiber:* The new labels are required to list fiber content, which will help people figure out if they are meeting their fiber goals. Currently, Americans consume 10 to 12 grams of fiber a day. Health authorities recommend 20 grams of fiber a day to stay "regular," which experts believe possibly prevents certain forms of cancer and other diseases.

- *Daily values*: These values show how a food fits into the overall daily diet. The daily values are based on a daily diet of 2,000 calories (individuals should adjust the values to fit their own calorie intake). The daily values provide figures for fat, saturated fat, cholesterol, sodium, carbohydrates, fiber, vitamins, and minerals.

- *New health claims:* Health claims on packaging will face stricter regulation. Food companies will now be allowed to illustrate seven relationships between a nutrient or a food and the risk of disease via statements, symbols (such as a heart), or descriptions. These relationships include: calcium and osteoporosis; fat and cancer; saturated fat and cholesterol and coronary heart disease; fiber-containing grain products, fruits, and vegetables and cancer; fruits, vegetables, and grain products that contain fiber and the risk of coronary heart disease; sodium and high blood pressure; and fruits and vegetables and cancer.

- *Ingredient changes:* Ingredient lists will be more specific. All color additives, rather than being referred to by the word "colors" will have to be specified by name. Sources of ingredients called protein hydrolysates will have to be listed by name rather than as "flavorings." This is good news for people following sodium-restricted diets because many of the protein hydrolysates are high in sodium. Beverages promoted as containing "juice" must state the exact percentage of juice present.

What's Not Included

- Levels of the B vitamins such as thiamin, riboflavin, and niacin will be omitted. Nutrient deficiencies are not the problem they were when the original label was developed. The new emphasis is on fat, cholesterol, sodium, and calories.

- Small packages: Any package smaller than 12 square inches (like a candy bar) does not have to provide nutrition information. It does need to include an address or phone number for consumer questions.

- Fat levels in infant's food: Labels on food for children under age two may not carry information related to calories from fat and saturated fat because the FDA wants to prevent parents from incorrectly assuming that infants and toddlers should restrict fat intake. Fat is important in the early development and growth years.

- Restaurant food, airline and cafeteria meals, ready-to-eat food prepared on site (bakery or deli), and food sold by mall and sidewalk vendors are exempt from nutrition labeling.

Label Literacy Lesson #2: The Label Table

Manufacturers may no longer use words such as light, reduced, and low fat however they choose. The FDA has mandated new definitions to describe these terms.

- **Free** means that a product contains no or only negligible amounts of fat, saturated fat, cholesterol, sodium, sugar, and/or calories.

- **Low** may be used on products that can be eaten frequently without a person exceeding the dietary guidelines for fat, saturated fat, cholesterol, sodium and/or calories. Specifically:

    —**Low fat**: 3 grams or fewer per serving

    —**Low saturated fat**: no more than 1 gram per serving

    —**Low sodium**: fewer than 140 milligrams per serving

    —**Low cholesterol**: fewer than 20 milligrams per serving

    —**Low calorie**: 40 calories or less per serving

- **Good source** means that one serving of a food contains 10 to 19 percent of the Daily Value for a particular nutrient.

- **High** indicates that a serving of food contains 20 percent more of the daily value for a specific nutrient.

- **Reduced** lets the customer know that a product has been nutritionally altered and contains 25 percent less of a nutrient or of calories than the regular product.

- **Less** indicates that a food contains 25 percent less of a nutrient or of calories than a comparable food. For example, pretzels could be labeled as containing 25 percent "less" fat than potato chips.

- Light means that the calories in a food product have been reduced by at least one third of what they were in the regular product, or that the fat is reduced by at least half. Light can also be used to refer to the texture and color of a food, however, the label must spell this out (for example, light brown sugar).

- **More** indicates that a serving of food contains at least 10 percent more of the daily value for a nutrient than the regular food.

- **Percent fat free** must now be used only on low fat or a fat-free products. The term is a reflection of the amount of the food's weight that is fat free. For example, if a serving of food weights 100 grams and two of the grams come from fat, it can be called "98 percent fat free."

- **Implied claims** such as "made with oat bran" or "no tropical oils" that mislead the consumer into believing a food does or does not contain significant amounts of certain nutrients are prohibited under the new labeling law. For instance, a manufacturer cannot claim that an item is made with oat bran unless it contains enough oat bran to meet the definition requirements for a "good source" of fiber. A claim that a product contains "no tropical oils" is allowed only on foods that are "low" in saturated fat because consumers have come to associate tropical oils with high saturated fat.

Calculating Percentage of Calories from Fat Using the New Food Label

The new label will include grams of fat and calories from fat. However, the percentage of calories from fat does not have to be listed.

Although some products will voluntarily include the percentage of calories from fat, you will need to calculate it on others.

Here's a simple formula for you to use:

Step #1. Take the calories from fat (per serving) and divide by the number of total calories per serving.

Step #2. Take this fraction and multiply by 100 to get the percentage of calories from fat.

For example, Lean Cuisine's new Turkey Pie contains 90 calories from fat and 310 total calories per serving.

Step #1.   90 divided by 310 = 0.29

Step #2.   0.29 times 100 = 29% calories from fat

A second example is Klondike Lite Ice Cream Sandwiches. They contain 18 calories from fat per serving and 90 total calories per serving.

Step #1.   18 divided by 90 = 0.20

Step #2.   0.20 times 100 = 20% calories from fat

Labels on Meat and Poultry Products

To make things even more complicated, a separate government agency, USDA's Food Safety and Inspection Service, approves food labeling on meat and poultry products. Manufacturers have until July 1994 to comply with the USDA labeling laws. Definitions for labeling terms commonly used on meat and poultry products are:

- **Free:** The product contains only a tiny or insignificant amount of fat, cholesterol, sodium, sugar, and/or calories. For example, a "fat-free" product will contains less than 0.5 grams of fat per serving.

- **Low**: A food described as low in fat, saturated fat, cholesterol, sodium, and/or calories could be eaten fairly often without exceeding dietary guidelines. So "low in fat" means no more than 3 grams of fat per serving.

- **Lean:** "Lean" and "Extra Lean" are USDA terms for use on meat and poultry products. "Lean" means the product contains less than 10 grams of fat, 4 grams of saturated fat, and 95 milligrams of cholesterol per serving. "Lean" is not as lean as "Low."

- **Extra Lean:** "Extra Lean" means the product has less than 5 grams of fat, 2 grams of saturated fat, and 95 milligrams of cholesterol per serving. "Extra Lean" is still not as lean as "Low."

- **Reduced, Less, Fewer:** Means a food product contains 25 percent less of a nutrient or calories. For example, hot dogs might be labeled "25% less fat than our regular hot dogs."

- **Light/Lite:** Means that a product has a third fewer calories or half the fat of the original. "Light in Sodium" means a product has half the usual amount of sodium.

- **More:** A food in which a serving has at least 10 percent more than usual of the daily value of a vitamin, mineral, or fiber.

- **Good Source Of:** One serving contains 10 to 19 percent of the daily value for a particular vitamin, mineral, or fiber.

Glossary of Old Labeling Terms

Here's the old glossary of terms so you can see how the labeling law has changed things. The list below indicates what the labels used to mean. Be alert, however, since some of these are still in effect.

Low Calories: 40 calories or less per serving and no more than 0.4 calories per gram. Foods naturally low in calories cannot be labeled low calorie. The FDA monitors whether the "serving size" chosen by the food company is reasonable.

Reduced Calorie: Must contain one-third less calories than the food it replaces and must include a comparison on the label.

Low Cholesterol: 20 milligrams or less per serving.

Reduced Cholesterol: Cannot contain more than one-fourth the cholesterol of the food it replaces.

No Cholesterol: No cholesterol is detectable by present analytical methods. (NOTE: These food items can still be high in fat!)

Cholesterol Free: Less than 2 milligrams cholesterol per serving. (Proposed by FDA.)

Diet or Dietetic: Same requirements as low or reduced calorie.

Enriched: This means that some, although not necessarily all, of the nutrients lost in food processing have been added back into the product.

Low Fat: Dairy products must contain between 0.5 and 2 percent milk fat to be labeled low-fat. Low-fat meat can be no more than 10 percent fat by weight.

Fortified: This means additional vitamins and minerals have been added during processing, such as vitamin D added to milk.

Hydrogenation: A process of adding hydrogen molecules to monounsaturated or polyunsaturated fatty acids. As a result, liquid oils chemically become more saturated (with hydrogen) and physically change from liquid to semisolid forms.

Imitation: Not the "real thing" and nutritionally inferior in that it is lower in protein, vitamins, or minerals.

"Lite" in general: Same definition as "low calorie" when "lite" refers to calorie content. (Companies could use the word "light" in advertising to refer to color or weight or whatever they want it to refer to, but not with the new law.)

Lower in fat: Has at least a 25 percent reduction in fat.

Natural or Organic: There is NO LEGAL DEFINITION, and there are no future plans by the FTC, FDA, or USDA to develop any.* Years ago these agencies met on this issue. The FTC agreed to take primary responsibility, but in 1983, it gave up on the task, saying they couldn't come up with a "suitable" definition. Suitable to whom, I wonder?

Salt-free, Unsalted: No salt was added to the product during processing, but it could contain significant sodium levels naturally or from other ingredients.

Very Low Sodium: 35 milligrams or less per serving.

Low Sodium: 140 milligrams or less per serving.

Reduced Sodium: The amount of sodium in the regular product is reduced by 75 percent.

Substitute: Not the "real thing" but nutritionally equivalent to the food it is imitating.

Sugar Free or Sugarless: These foods cannot contain sucrose (table sugar) but can have other sweeteners, including honey, corn syrup, fructose, sorbitol, etc.

---

* Guess which state managed to come up with its very own definition in 1981 for "organic" and "organically grown?" California, of course! Through the California Sherman Food, Drug, and Cosmetic Law of the Department of Health Services.

The Ingredient Label

Under Federal law, all food products must list the ingredients starting with the ingredient added in the largest quantity (by weight) and continuing in descending order. So, if you want a general idea of what you'll be eating, check out the first three or four ingredients. With the new labeling law, ingredient lists will be even more specific. You'll want to reread the section above on these changes. But for now, let's take a little quiz about ingredients. I'll list the first four ingredients of a popular food and you guess what food it is:

Quiz:
Would you put this in your mouth?

1. Carbonated water, high fructose corn syrup and/or sucrose, caramel color, phosphoric acid.

2. Soybean oil, partially hydrogenated soybean oil, whole eggs, vinegar.

3. Sugar, enriched wheat flour, vegetable and animal shortening (partially hydrogenated soybean oil, hydrogenated cottonseed oil, lard), cocoa.

4. Water, corn syrup, hydrogenated coconut and palm kernel oils, sugar.

5. Milk chocolate (sugar, milk, cocoa butter, chocolate, lecithin, vanillin—an artificial flavor), peanuts, corn syrup, sugar.

6. Sugar, citric acid, potassium citrate (regulates tartness).

7. Soybean oil, water, sugar.

8. Sugar, partially hydrogenated animal and/or vegetable shortening, enriched flour.

9. Milled and flaked corn, salt, sugar.

10. Enriched corn meal, vegetable oil (contains 1 or more of the following: Cottonseed oil, corn oil, peanut oil, partially hydrogenated cot-

tonseed oil, partially hydrogenated soybean oil, partially hydrogenated sunflower oil or palm oil), whey.

11.   Corn syrup, brown sugar, peanut butter.

12.   Pork snouts, cured pork tongues, water.

13.   Water, sugar and corn syrups, fruit juices and purees.

Answers:

1. Coke, 2. Mayonnaise, 3. Oreo Cookies, 4. Cool Whip, 5. Snickers Candy Bar, 6. Tang, 7. Kraft Thousand Island Dressing, 8. HoHo Snack Cakes, 9. Shake & Bake, pork flavor, 10. Chee-tos Cheese Twists, 11. Tiger's Milk Nutrition Bar (original protein-rich flavor), 12. Head cheese cold cut, 13. Hawaiian Punch (in ready-to-drink boxes)

Some foods have standard ingredients, such as jellies, jams, ketchup, ice cream, mayonnaise, peanut butter, cheeses, and milk, and are not required to list the ingredients. Unfortunately, sometimes these products contain ingredients some people could be allergic to, but they still don't need to be listed. When these foods are made "lighter," you'll notice they usually get called something else such as "sandwich spread" instead of mayonnaise or "Light Dessert" instead of ice cream.

Label Literacy Lesson #3

• **Beware of Ingredients That Are What They Don't Appear to Be**

Sometimes we think we can outsmart the food companies by reading our labels solely for that nasty word "sugar." But remember, those guys make it their business (and a big profit-making business at that) to always stay a few steps ahead of the consumer. So, let's get ahead of the game.

Sugar (refined carbohydrate, processed sugar, etc.) goes by many names, none significantly better than the others. The aliases include:

Sucrose	Dextrose
Fructose	Honey
Brown sugar	High fructose corn syrup
Maltose	Molasses
Invert sugar	

Syrups (for example, corn or maple syrup)

"Sweeteners" (for example, corn sweeteners)

Sodium in disguise

Hard to imagine, but more than 70 sodium-containing substances are added to foods today. Salt (sodium chloride) leads the pack. "Sodium" and "salt" are used interchangeably. Here are some of the sodium-containing criminals:

Salt (sodium chloride), the major sodium contributor in the American diet. Salt is 40 percent sodium.

MSG (monosodium glutamate)

Soy sauce

Brine (salt and water)

Broth and bouillon

Sodium compounds:

>   Sodium phosphate
>
>   Sodium benzoate
>
>   Sodium bicarbonate (baking soda)
>
>   Sodium hydroxide
>
>   Sodium propionate
>
>   Sodium sulfite
>
>   Baking powder

And any other compounds with the word "sodium" in them.

Fats also come in disguises:

Butter

All oils, such as vegetable, coconut, palm kernel, etc.

Shortening, vegetable or animal

Hydrogenated fats or oils

Animal fats, such as bacon or pork fat, beef fat, lard, suet, chicken or turkey fat

Mono- or diglycerides

Glycerolesters

Cocoa butter, chocolate, or milk chocolate

Cream

Egg and egg-yolk solids

Whole-milk solids

Taking a Tour Through Your Supermarket

Picture yourself sandwiched between a shopping cart and a conglomeration of salad dressing bottles. Which dressing do you grab? You want to reduce the fat in your diet, but you don't even know where to start. Where's a nutritionist when you need one? Similar problems can strike as you cruise the cracker aisle or face countless fancy-named entrees in the frozen food section. You can't even buy cat food these days without dealing with a cloud of brands and flavors—most, for some reason, with fancier names than people food.

So, if I can't accompany you on a trip through your supermarket, you can tag along through mine, as I hopefully answer some of your questions. (I won't even attempt to answer cat food questions. But then we all know who really "chooses" the flavor and brand anyway.)

The Frozen Food Aisles

Given the invitation to give up half my refrigerator space for an equal amount of expansion in the freezer compartment, I would gladly accept. I attribute this love of freezer space not only to my over-reliance on freezing individualized portions of leftovers in plastic containers but also to several fabulous frozen foods I've found over the years.

Frozen Bagels

Sounds simple, I know, but you might consider their value one morning when you only have two minutes to fix your breakfast. This is exactly the amount of time it takes to split your frozen bagel in half, pop it in the toaster, prepare the filling for when the bagel pops up, wrap it in a napkin, and go! Bagels, by themselves, are low in fat, so they can be a great snack or breakfast on the run.

Egg Substitutes

While we're on the subject of breakfast, I'll mention another favorite frozen food find—frozen eggs. But not just any frozen eggs—Fleischmann's Egg Beaters. As far as I can tell, they were the first to come out with a cholesterol-free egg substitute that was also fat free! Since then many of the others companies reformulated their egg substitutes to be equally as low fat or fat free. Egg Beaters is 99 percent egg white (remember all the fat and cholesterol in eggs are in the yolk), which explains why it has almost no fat (about 4 calories from fat) and very few calories (25 per 1/4 cup). It looks like scrambled eggs so you can use it in omelettes, quiche, and so on.

What About Frozen Breakfast Foods?

You can now buy everything from breakfast muffins to a complete egg, sausage, and hash browns breakfast in the frozen food section. The egg and sausage type selections don't even come close to meeting my diet guidelines, and neither do the croissant varieties, no matter how whole-wheaty and "au naturel" they make them sound.

Ms. Sara Lee, for example, labels her "Healthy Fruit Muffins" as FIBER RICH, but she's not telling just how much fiber these little babies actually contain. This isn't surprising considering sugar ranks as the first ingredient in this product.

If you're a frozen pancake lover and you've joined the wave of microwave users, you can choose from several different brands: All the breakfast-type products that meet the guidelines are listed on the following chart.:

Frozen Breakfast Products

Item	Serving Size	Calories	% Calories from Fat	Fat (gms)	Sodium (mg)
Kellogg's					
Special K Waffles	1	80	0	0	130
Belgian					
Chef Waffles	1	70	13%	1.25	170
Aunt Jemima					
Low-fat Waffles	1	80	<11%	1	270
Krusteaz					
Mini Pancakes	6	120	15%	2	280
French Toast					
Cinnamon	2 slices	250	22%	6	600
Classic Style	4 oz.	250	22%	6	380
Pancakes					
Blueberry	3	280	16%	5	710
Buttermilk	3	290	15.5%	3	740
Swanson					
Breakfast Blast–mini pancakes w/syrup	6	300	24%	8	580
Breakfast Blast –mini French Toast w/syrup	4	180	25%	5	190
Weight Watchers					
English Muffin s/w	1	240	30%	8	540
Handy Ham & Cheese Omelet	1	240	30%	8	540
Ham & Cheese Bagel	1	210	26%	6	450
Classic Omelette	1	210	30%	7	410
Garden Omelette	1	210	26%	6	480
Banana Nut Muffins	2.5 oz	170	26%	5	250
Cinnamon Streusel Coffee Cakes	2.25 oz	160	22.5%	4	190
Harvest Honey Bran Muffins	1 oz	160	22.5%	4	150

Now that you've bought a frozen breakfast that meets the guidelines and you're heating it up, are you going to add gobs of butter or whipped cream? Absolutely not! But you can add whatever fruit you want, such as sliced or baked apples, peaches, or frozen berries. Any fresh fruit will go great on top of a waffle, pancake, or slice of french toast. A modest amount (2 tablespoons on a stack of three pancakes) of "lite" or flavored syrup can also be added.

Frozen Entrees

Dinner recipes have a tough challenge ahead—it's not enough anymore simply to taste good or to be "gourmet." Dinner recipes today compete head on with meals that can be popped in the microwave and ready to eat in eight to ten minutes. Americans everywhere have enthusiastically discovered the "frozen entree."

In the next few pages, though, we're only going to talk about the "light" entrees, since they're the only ones that have nutrition information on the packaging. Remember, when a company makes a nutritional claim about their product, such as saying it's "lite" or "low calorie," legally the nutrition information must be on the label along with the mandatory list of ingredients.

The distinguished list of contenders includes Le Menu, Light Style, Healthy Choice by Con Agra, Tyson-Gourmet Slim Selects, Lean Cuisine, and Weight Watchers. Notice the buzz words "slim," "lean," "weight." All these enticing descriptors are based solely on calories—not FAT. This falsely impressive "low-calorie" status is not accomplished through anything terribly magical or scientific. This is an exercise in good old-fashioned portion control! The smaller the portion, the lower the calories.

For our purposes—for fighting FAT—we won't be judging frozen entrees merely on their caloric contributions. We're going to up the ante and factor in fat, following these five rules for healthy eating.

Rule # 1: No Info, No Purchase

If you can't find the number of calories and grams of fat printed on the package, don't buy it! You need to know this information before making a decision about whether to eat this unknown food.

Rule #2: The 25 Percent Solution

Make sure you start out with an entree that contains 25 percent or less calories from fat. Most entree labels will list the calories per serving and grams of fat. From this you will need to figure out the percent of calories from fat. To do this, multiply grams of fat per serving by 9—the number of calories per gram of fat. Then convert this to a percentage by dividing by the number of calories per serving and multiplying by 100.

Next time you stock up on frozen entrees, bring a calculator with you. That way you can calculate the percent of calories from fat as you walk down the aisle deciding which ones to try. Here's a list of the entrees I found with less than 30 percent of calories from FAT:

Frozen Entrees

Food Item	Calories	Fat (gm)	% Fat Calories	Sodium (mg)
Weight Watchers				
Broccoli & Cheese Baked Potato	230	7	27%	510
Cheese Tortellini	310	6	17%	570
Fettucini Alfredo with Broccoli	230	7	27%	550
Garden Lasagna	260	7	24%	430
Italian Cheese Lasagna	290	7	22%	510
Macaroni & Cheese	280	6	19%	550
Beef Enchiladas Rancheros	190	5	24%	500
Chicken Cordon Bleu	170	5	26%	560
Chicken Kiev	190	5	24%	470
Grilled Glazed Chicken	180	5	25%	300
London Broil in Mushroom Sauce	110	3	24.5%	320
Oven-Baked Fish	140	3	19%	370

Food Item	Calories	Fat (gm)	%Fat Calories	Sodium (mg)
Teriyaki Chicken with Sauce	150	4	24%	590
Veal Patty Parmigiana	150	4	24%	550
Weight Watchers Smart Ones				
Chicken Francais	150	1	6%	400
Chicken Mirabella	160	1	5.5%	420
Fiesta Chicken	210	1	4%	390
Lasagna Florentine	221	1	4%	460
Pasta Portafino	160	1	5.6%	220
Weight Watchers Stir-Fry				
Jade Garden Beef	150	3	18%	490
Sesame Chicken with Lo Mein Noodles	200	4	18%	420
Banquet Healthy Balance				
Chicken Parmesan Meal	300	9	27%	800
Turkey & Gravy Meal with Dressing	270	5	17%	750
The Budget Gourmet				
Glazed Turkey	260	5	17%	710
Mandarin Chicken	250	5	18%	550
Orange Glazed Chicken Breast	270	3	10%	870
Roast Chicken with Homestyle Gravy	210	7	30%	690
Italian Style Vegetables and Chicken	310	8	23%	690
Stuffed Turkey Breast	250	6	22%	570
Macaroni & Cheese with Cheddar and Parmesan	330	8	22%	760
Teriyaki chicken	280	7	22.5%	460
Le Menu American Cuisine				
Old Fashioned Pot Roast	230	7	27%	570
Healthy Choice				
Breast of Turkey	260	3	10%	560
Salisbury Steak	280	6	19%	500
Sirloin Tips	270	7	23%	360
Sweet & Sour Chicken	300	4	12%	230
Yankee Pot Roast	260	4	14%	400
Chicken & Vegetables	280	3	10%	380

Food Item	Calories	Fat (gm)	%Fat Calories	Sodium (mg)
Chicken Low Mein	220	3	12%	440
Chicken Fettucini	240	4	15%	370
Chicken or Beef Enchiladas	320	6	17%	550
Chicken or Beef Fajitas	200	3	13.5%	310
Glazed Chicken	220	3	12%	510
Herb Chicken	380	7	16.5%	470
Lasagna	260	5	17%	420
Mesquite Chicken	350	4	10%	380
Nacho Macaroni & Cheese	280	5	16%	560
Roast Turkey with Mushroom Gravy	200	3	13.5%	380
Salsa Chicken Dinner	240	2	7.5%	450
Seasoned Beef Ribs with BBQ Sauce	330	6	16%	530
Sliced Turkey with Gravy and Dressing	270	4	13%	530
Teriyaki Chicken with Pasta	350	3	8%	370

Lean Cuisine (Stouffer's)

Food Item	Calories	Fat (gm)	%Fat Calories	Sodium (mg)
Beef & Bean Enchaladas	240	6	22.5%	480
Beef Cannelloni	200	3	13.5%	490
Breast of Chicken & Herbs	240	5	19%	490
Breast of Chicken Marsala	180	4	20%	430
Chicken a l'Orange	280	4	13%	290
Chicken Chow Mein	240	5	19%	530
Chicken in BBQ Sauce	260	6	21%	500
Chicken in Peanut Sauce	290	7	22%	530
Chicken Italiano	290	8	25%	490
Chicken Oriental	280	7	22.5%	480
Chicken with Vegetables	240	5	19%	500
Fiesta Chicken	240	5	19%	560
Homestyle Turkey	230	5	19.5%	550
Lasagna	280	6	19%	560
Angel Hair Pasta	240	5	19%	410
Fettucini Alfredo	280	7	22.5%	570
Fettucini Primavera	260	7	24%	580
Macaroni & Beef	250	6	22%	540

Food Item	Calories	Fat (gm)	%Fat Calories	Sodium (mg)
Sliced Turkey Breast in Mushroom Sauce	230	7	27%	540
Spaghetti with Meatballs	290	7	22%	550
Stuffed Cabbage	210	6	26%	560
Swedish Meatballs	290	8	25%	550
Turkey Dijon	210	6	26%	590
Zucchini Lasagna	260	5	17%	550
Lean Cuisine Lunch Express				
Cheese Lasagna Casserole	290	6	19%	560
Mandarin Chicken	270	5	17%	570
Teriyaki Stir Fry	260	5	17%	510
Fettucini with Chicken in Alfredo Sauce	240	6	22.5%	540
Oriental Style Stir Fry	280	7	22.5%	590
Pasta with Chicken in Herb Tomato Sauce	270	6	20%	460
Michelina's				
Spaghetti Marinara	255	2	7%	681
Tyson				
Chicken Mesquite	320	8	22.5%	660
Chicken Marsala	180	3	15%	600
Chicken Picata	200	4	18%	550
Tyson Healthy Portion				
Mesquite Chicken Meal	330	5	14%	600
Honey Mustard Chicken Meal	390	6	14%	520

Maybe you already have a favorite frozen entree—one you salivate over while driving home from work. Even though they have diet-like names, you still need to process the nutrient data for yourself. Some of these inno-cent looking and sounding entrees are actually way over 30 percent of calo-ries from fat.

Rule #3: Cutting the FAT

If that favorite entree of yours is more than 25 percent calories from fat but less than 30 percent, relax. You can still work it out. When you balance the meal by adding any missing complex carbohydrates (rule #4 below), the total meal will come down to 25 percent of calories from fat.

Rule #4: Finding the Missing Carbohydrates

Check the entree for missing complex carbohydrates by running through the complex carbohydrate roll call: Vegetables, Fruits, Grains, Starches, Cereals. Work these foods into the meal. If the entree doesn't come with a vegetable, add some to it. Sometimes you can just stir them right into the entree, like with Chicken a l'Orange or Oriental Style Shrimp with Rice.

Using frozen entrees may require a teeny bit of planning. You may need to prepare or bring along whatever complex carbohydrate you need to complete the meal. Two examples are:

- If you bring a Zucchini Lasagna (Lean Cuisine) to work for lunch, pack an orange or apple and a roll with it in the morning.
- If you have Fillet of Fish Divan for dinner, boil some rice or noodles while your entree is cooking. (It already has broccoli.) Cut up some melon or strawberries to add the missing complex carbohydrates.

Rule #5: Hide the Salt Shaker

Salt has already been added—sometimes in massive amounts, I might add—to your frozen entrees. So adding more salt at the table is a major no-no.

Ice Cream, You Scream

I'm one of those people who, if given a nudge or two, could eat ice cream every day. Double chocolate fudge, strawberry delight, virtuous vanilla—it really doesn't matter which, as long as it's ice cream. This wonderful multi-season treat addicts people with its "light yet creamy" feeling, comes in oh-so-many-fun-flavors, and tops a meal or warm Sunday afternoon like no other.

You might think I'm setting you up with images of ice cream just to let you down with healthful horror stories. Would a fellow ice cream lover do that? Actually, I'm happy to announce that lower fat selections in the frozen dessert aisle have never looked better: Gone are the days of only chocolate or vanilla ice milk. Say hello to mint chocolate chip, mocha nut sundae, and strawberry cheesecake—and that's just the first couple rows!

I took to the ice cream section with clipboard and calculator in hand, writing down only those items with less than 30 percent of calories from fat—which usually means 8 grams or less of fat per 1-cup serving. But to help you truly appreciate the significance of these great lower fat options, let's review what the regular rich ice creams would add. The standard store brand ice cream has around 300 calories per cup, 48 percent from fat, and the fancy rich types can add from 400 to 600 calories per cup, with up to 60 percent of calories from fat. Even sherbets have up to 300 calories per cup because the calories they don't have from cream are present in sugar. A better choice would be the fruit sorbets, sweetened with mostly fruit juice instead of plain old sugar.

Now for the good news:

The following items contain no more than 25 percent calories from fat, 2 grams or less fat per 3-ounce serving, and do not have sucrose or other sugars listed as the first or second ingredient (besides water).

Ice Cream

Brand	Grams of fat per 1/2 cup	Calories	% Calories from fat
Knudsen Nice N'Light			
Chocolate			
Chocolate Marble			
Neopolitan			
Strawberry Swirl			
Chocolate Chip			
Cookies & Cream	2-3	100-120	18-22%
Healthy Choice	2	120	15%
Check labels; new flavors appear daily!			

Brand	Grams of Fat per 1/2 cup	Calories	% Calories from fat
Dreyers Grand Light (Vanilla)	4	100	36%
Breyers Light (Vanilla)	4	120	30%
Baskin Robbins 31			
Fat Free Just Peachy	0	100	0
Light Strawberry Royal	3	110	24.5%
Light Double Chocolate	3	110	24.5%

Frozen Yogurt

Brand	Grams of Fat per 1/2 cup	Calories	% Calories from fat
Honey Hill Farms			
Soft Style	1	130	7%
Colombo			
Shoppe Style Soft Low-fat Frozen Yogurt Most Flavors (except Peanut Butter Twist)	1 (per 3 oz.)	90	10%
Dreyers Frozen Yogurt Inspirations			
(Boysenberry Vanilla Swirl, Marble Fudge, Orange Vanilla Swirl)	3	100-110	25-27%
Vanilla Chocolate Swirl	0	90	0
Chocolate	0	90	0
Banana Strawberry	0	80	0
Raspberry	0	90	0
Vanilla	0	90	0
Dannon Light Frozen Yogurt			
(Peach, Vanilla, Chocolate, Cherry Vanilla Swirl)	<1	80-90	10%

Lower Fat Dairy Products:
Pass the low-fat milk, please!*

Where would most meals and beverages be without milk? It's still the best thing for lightening your coffee—better than cream and nondairy creamers. (Most of the latter still have the same amount of FAT as cream— just not the cholesterol.) We need milk to keep our cereal company, wet our pancake batters, and on and on. But along with bringing all these attributes to our table, it brings fat calories and cholesterol.

The great thing about milk, though, is you can "skim" some (low-fat milk) or most (nonfat milk) of the fat away and still have a milk that, for the most part, does all the things you want it to do. And the other amazing trick with milk is as the fat calories decrease, so does the cholesterol. Actually this is true of most foods with fat, since cholesterol goes where the fat is. As you remove the fat, you are also removing the cholesterol.

They say seeing is believing. Listed below are the average nutrient values from the assorted ways to buy your milk, starting with the lowest in fat and moving to the highest. Remember to watch the cholesterol go up, too.

	Calories per 1 Cup	% fat calories	Fat (gm)	Cholesterol (mg)
Skim milk	86	5	0.4	5
Buttermilk	99	20	2.0	7
Low-fat milk (1% milkfat)	102	22	2.5	14
Low-fat milk (2% milkfat)	121	35	4.8	22
Whole milk (3.3% milkfat)	150	49	8.0	34

---

* This information applies only to people over the age of two. Children under age two need the fat and fat soluble vitamins of whole milk because of their rapid rate of growth and development.

Cottage Cheese

Low-fat cottage cheese is certainly not one of the more glamorous dairy products on the market today. But it quite possibly could have the most promising future amidst the rising low-fat furor in America.

I'm asking you to look beyond the "diet food" stereotype that has haunted cottage cheese over the years. You know the one—the tortuous diet plate featuring a boring white mound of cottage cheese sitting on a pineapple ring (and if you're lucky, a cherry on top).

No, what I've got in store for cottage cheese today and beyond is a whole lot more exciting. Fancy cottage cheese whipped with Philadelphia Light Cream Cheese with a bit of pesto layered on top for a tasty colorful spread. Picture whipped cottage cheese as an extender for your favorite frosting. Imagine a cup of cottage cheese whipped with only a couple tablespoons of reduced-calorie mayonnaise to make a creamy potato or pasta salad. And that's only the beginning!

I've been experimenting with cottage cheese lately and am finding out the only limit to composing new uses for cottage cheese is my own imagination. I mean, what could I have been thinking when I mixed half the usual amount of vanilla frosting with the same amount of whipped nonfat cottage cheese? (You can "whip" cottage cheese and smooth out the lumps by using a food processor or blender.) But you know, it actually worked. People didn't even notice the difference! I've even started using half cottage cheese (whipped) and half light cream cheese to make a lower fat cheesecake.

If low-fat cottage cheese isn't low fat enough for you, progress has already visited the cottage cheese case. Knudsen introduced NONFAT cottage cheese as part of their new "Nice 'N Light" line.

When cottage cheese is whipped in a food processor or blender, it transforms into something resembling ricotta cheese. And today's low and nonfat cottage cheese options make it a lower fat filler to your favorite pasta dishes, a lower fat thickener for creamy sauces, and the major ingredient of choice for dips and creamy dressings.

Just so you can appreciate the value of this truly momentous dairy discovery, in the following table I've listed calories, fat, and cholesterol content of the new nonfat cottage cheese alongside the fattier ingredients it can replace.

	Calories per 1/2 cup	% Calories from Fat	Cholesterol (mg)	Sodium (mg)
Knudsen Nonfat Cottage Cheese	70	5%	6	420
Low-fat Cottage Cheese (2%)	102	20%	10	459

Items that can be replaced by cottage cheese:

	Calories per 1/2 cup	% Calories from fat	Cholesterol (mg)	Sodium (mg)
Part-skim ricotta cheese	170	53%	40	154
Regular sour cream	247	36%	64	57
Knudsen Light Sour Cream	180	60%	not listed	100
Best Foods Light Reduced Calorie Mayonnaise	400	91%	78	624
Regular mayonnaise	788	98%	78	624
Regular cream cheese	396	88%	124	336
Light Philadelphia (tub)	240	75%	not listed	160

Say "Cheese"

One of our favorite foods is cheese. Whether it sits on a cracker, tops our tortilla, or is layered in our lasagna, let's face it, we love cheese! Unfortunately, cheeses are "fat city." You can cut your fat per ounce almost in half by buying the reduced fat (part skim type) cheeses. Who can refuse an offer like that?

"Reduced fat" cheeses should have no more than 5 grams of fat per ounce. The following items meet this guideline:

Alpine Lace–American Cheese Slices

Bordens Lite Line Singles–All flavors

Cracker Barrel Light–Sharp Cheddar

Frigo–Truly Lite Mozzarella, String Cheese

Kraft—Free Singles, Light Singles, Vermont Sharp White Cheddar

Laughing Cow Reduced Calorie Cheese–Bonbel

Lifetime Cheese–Cheddar, Monterey Jack, Swiss

Nob Hill Light–Monterey Jack

Polly-O–Lite Part-Skim Mozzarella

Precious–Lite Mozzarella

Sargento–Light Mozzarella, Shredded

Smartbeat (No Cholesterol)–American Slices

Velveeta–Velveeta Light

Weight Watchers–Mild Cheddar, Monterey Jack, Shredded Cheddar, Sharp Cheddar, Sharp Cheddar Processed Cheese Slices, American Singles, Low Sodium American Singles

Other cheese products with at least one-third less fat than the regular items:

Soft cheeses and sour creams

Brand	Calories per serving	% Calories from fat	Fat (gm)	Cholesterol (mg)	Sodium (mg)
Frigo Truly Lite Fat-Free Ricotta	20	0	0	3	15
Frigo Truly Lite Low-fat Low Salt	30	30%	1		10
Precious Low Fat	40	48%	2	10	20
Cream Cheeses Light Philadelphia Block	70	77%	6	20	115
Light Philadelphia Tub	60	75%	5	10	160
Philadelphia Free	25	0	0	5	170
Sour Creams Healthy Choice Fat Free	30	0	0	5	200
Knudsen Free	18	0	0	0	20
Knudsen Light	35	51%	2	10	20
Real Dairy No Fat	15	0	0	0	15
Land 'O Lakes Light	40	45%	2		25
Land 'O Lakes No Fat Cholesterol Free Sour Cream Substitute	50	72%	4	0	40

Processed Meat Items

I went on a processed meats section expedition a couple of years ago in search of healthful items and found almost nothing worth mentioning. But now, I can even buy a lower fat hot dog! Now, that's progress. After this year's investigation (reading labels), I was so excited about the positive changes I had seen that I took home some "Less Fat" turkey franks and surprised my husband that night with hot dogs and fries (they were low-fat fries, of course). He thought he was in the wrong house.

The following are the lunch meats I found that are actually "low in fat," having less than 30 percent of their calories from fat:

Lunch meats

Brand	Calories	Fat (gm)	Sodium (mg)
	Per 1 oz. serving		
Healthy Choice			
Oven Roasted Turkey Breast	30	1	285
Baked Ham	35	1	260
Oven Roasted Chicken Breast	35	1	300
Honey Ham	30	1	280
Smoked Turkey	30	1	240
Butterball Fresh Deli			
Smoked Chicken Breast	30	0.5	240
Smoked Turkey Breast	30	0.5	240
Honey Roasted and Smoked Turkey Breast	35	1	235
Oven Roasted Turkey Breast	30	1	285
Hillshire Farms Deli Select			
Smoked Turkey Breast	30	0.5	305
Honey Roasted Turkey Breast	30	<0.5	270
Louis Rich			
Oven Roasted Turkey Breast	25	<1	320
Hickory Smoked Turkey Breast	25	<1	280
Turkey Pastrami	25	<1	260
Deli-Thin Oven Roasted Turkey Breast	30	<2.5	312.5

Brand	Calories	Fat (gm)	Sodium (mg)
	Per 1 oz. serving		
Danola Danish Ham	30	1	NA
Oscar Mayer			
Roasted Turkey Breast, Thin Sliced	32	0.7	364
Baked Cooked Ham Slices	27	<1.5	337
Smoked Turkey Breast Slices	20	<1.5	337
Smoked Cooked Ham	27	<1.5	378
Oscar Mayer Healthy Favorites Deli Thin (per slice)			
Oven Roasted Turkey Breast	28	<2	307
Honey Ham	33	<2	307
Oven Roasted Chicken	12	<2	260

Other Boxes, Bottles, and Cans

Cereal

Most of us ate it for the first time long before our first birthday. And some of us, now deep into adulthood, remain faithful cereal eaters. Whether you prefer it hot, wet, or dry, most everyone likes some type of cereal. And we all eat it our own special way—letting the cereal sit in the milk for just the right amount of time, munching it right out of the box, or anything you like.

We develop our own little cereal rituals because we've had so much practice. (Only after eating the last marshmallow Lucky Charm, for example, would I turn to the wheaty loops.) If you figure that most of us, as children, ate cereal at least five times a week, that means we sat down to a bowl of cereal about 2,400 times in 10 years.

The word "cereal" traces back to the Latin word "Ceres," the Romen goddess of agriculture and corn. However, the story goes, the word "cereal" sprang forth from humble grainy beginnings. But long after the Roman empire, assorted goddesses, and ancient crops of wheat, rye, and corn, cereal became a big American business. Breakfast grains are now processed, colored, sugar-coated (sometimes sliced with oil), packaged, and then promoted. Some are touted by Tigers named Tony, others by serious sounding people relaying serious quotes from the National Cancer Institute.

Considering the small amount of talent and time it takes to prepare a bowl of cereal, you can bet the cereal market isn't going anywhere but up. It then becomes extra important to buy the box that will *contribute* to good health—rather than threaten it.

As any of you cereal lovers, or parents of cereal lovers, can attest, the cereal aisle is full of colors, confusion, and what seems like hundreds of choices. The good news is the nutrition information provided on cereal labels has improved greatly. Today, in most cases, the grams of dietary fiber per serving along with the carbohydrate grams from "sucrose and other sugars" are listed.

To find out what percentage of the calories are from sucrose and other sugars, follow these steps:

Step 1:   Multiply the grams listed for "Sucrose and Other Sugars" per serving by 4. (You will always multiply this number by 4 because there are 4 calories per gram of carbohydrate.)

Step 2:   Divide this new number by the total calories listed per serving.

Step 3:   Multiply by 100 to get the percent.

Just so the suspense doesn't keep you up tonight and ruin tomorrow's breakfast, here's what I deduced after my last journey through the cereal jungle.

Cereals with 4 grams or more fiber

Per 1 1/2-cup serving (unless otherwise noted)

Cereal	Fiber (gm)	Calories	Fat (gms)	Sodium (mg)	% Calories from sugar
All Bran with extra fiber, 2/3 cup	28	100	0	280	0
Bran Chex	13.5	234	2	681	18%
Fruit & Fibre, Peaches/Almonds	11	269	4.5	381	17%
Fruit & Fibre, Dates/Walnuts	11	269	4.5	381	17%

Cereal	Fiber (gms)	Calories	Fat (gms)	Sodium (mg)	% Calories from sugar
Most	9.7	262	1	412	24%
Shredded Wheat 'N Bran	9	202	1	0	0
Shredded Wheat with Oat Bran	9	224	2.2	0	0
Kellogg's 40% Bran Flakes	8	190	1	453	22%
Grapenuts, 3/4 cup	7.2	304	0.4	594	12%
Shredded Wheat, Small	7	228	1.4	6	3%
Frosted Mini-Wheats, 8-9 biscuits	7	224	0	0	24%
Common Sense Oat Bran	6	200	2	520	24%
Quaker Oat Bran	6	200	4	250	16%
Quaker Oat Bran Squares	6	300	3	405	24%
Muesli, Apple/Almond, 1 cup	6	300	4	280	13%
Muesli, Almond/Date, 1 cup	6	280	4	190	14%
Post Raisin Bran, 1.4 oz.	6	120	1	200	23%
Wheat Chex	5	252	1.7	462	7%
Wheaties	4.5	152	0.7	414	11%
Just Right with Fiber Nuggets	4.5	224	2.2	440	20%
Whole Wheat Total	4.5	150	1.5	300	12%
NutriGrain Wheat	4.2	237	0.7	448	7%

Low-fat cereals with less than 4 grams of fiber

Per 1 1/2 cup Serving (unless otherwise noted)

Cereal	Fiber (gms)	Calories	Fat (gms)	Sodium (mg)	% Calories from Sugar
Cheerios	2	110	2	290	4%
Rice Chex	NA	110	0	240	7%
Kellogg's Cornflakes	1	100	0	290	8%
Triples	NA	110	1	200	8%
Corn Chex	NA	110	0	280	11%
Total Corn Flakes	NA	110	<1	200	11%
Rice Krispies	0	110	0	290	11%
Crispix	1	11-	0	220	11%
Kix	NA	110	<1	260	11%
Wheat Chex	3	100	1	230	12%
Multigrain Cheerios	2	100	1	230	24%
Frosted Mini Wheats	3	100	0	0	24%
Life	2	100	2	150	24%
Quaker Puffed Rice	0	100	0	0	0
Quaker Puffed Wheat	2	100	0	0	0
NutriGrain Raisin Bran	5	130	1	290	7%
NutriGrain Almond/Raisin	3	140	2	220	13%
Ralston Sun Flakes	0	110	1	240	0
Special K	1	110	0	230	0
Grapenuts Flakes	3	100	1	140	9%

See, that's not so bad, is it? If you want to know the calories per serving or if you are wondering why your favorite cereal isn't on these lists, check the nutrition label on the box. Some cereals could have been left off because they're too new or not available in Northern California, where I read my labels.

Cereal box reading could become your new hobby. You might discover some of the real healthy sounding cereals have over a third of their calories from sugars, and there are certain words to stay away from, such as "frosted" and "fruity." I also found that when some perfectly great bran or grain cereals make a new variation like "cinnamon" or "with raisins" they end up adding other items (namely sugars or more fat). Guess where all this put Tony the Tiger and the Trix rabbit. In the dog house!

Crackers

Most of us know that crackers tend to be loaded down with fat and salt. But that doesn't mean we never find ourselves buying crackers. A lot of the spreads we cover our crackers with are also high in fat, sodium, and who knows what else. So we want to make sure, at least, that we start out with a low-fat (less than 30 percent of calories from fat), low-salt cracker, right?

And the final contestants for the "low-fat" (sometimes "lower sodium") crackers category are:

Low-fat Crackers

Per 1 ounce serving

Brand	Calories	% Calories from fat	Fat (gm)	Sodium (mg)
SnackWell's				
Cracked Pepper	120	0	0	320
Fat Free Cinnamon Graham	100	0	0	90
Reduced Fat Cheese Crackers				
Fat Free Wheat Crackers	100	0	0	320
Mister Salty				
Fat Free Pretzel Chips	100	0	0	620
Lightly Salted Pretzel Chips	120	0	2	400
Original Pretzel Chips	120	0	2	620
Nabisco				
Premium Fat Free (1/2 oz.)	100	0	0	230
Zwieback	120	15%	2	40
Natural Rye Krisp				
Regular	80	0		150
Seasoned	90	20%	2	210
Old London Melba Toast				
Rye	100	<18	<2	210
White	100	<18	<2	220
Wasa				
Hearty Rye	100	0		150
Lite Rye	86	0		136
Golden Rye	92	0		130
Kavli Norwegian				
Thick Flat	120		<3	120

Jams, Jellies, and Preserves—
An Alternative to Fats

Many of us have said no to jams and jellies for years because we know they're usually laced with sugar or corn syrup—most of the time with only a little more fruit than sugar. But let me try and make a case for the fine preserves out there.

When do we usually dip into that jar of jam? How about just after we toasted an English muffin or bagel? Okay. So what could we coat our bread with instead? Remember, butter, cream cheese, etc., are all high in calories and the percentage of calories from fat.

Let's put it this way. Say you toast an English muffin and instead of margarine, you grab the Smucker's low-sugar boysenberry spread. Your snack just became respectable. It went from 237 calories to 150 and from 47 percent of calories from fat to 6 percent of calories from fat.

All right, so maybe you're not into nooks and crannies. Maybe you're more the bagel type—slicing an ounce or two of cream cheese in the middle. Using 2 tablespoons of a low-sugar type of jam or preserve instead will save you about 50 calories and will transform your fatty breakfast from 39 percent of calories from fat to 6 percent! And that's just switching to a reduced sugar preserve. There are all types of NO sugar preserves in your market, too. (Once you open the jar, these tend to spoil faster. So if you're the only jam eater in your house, you might want to buy the smaller-sized jars.)

	Calories	% Calories from Fat	% Protein	% Carbohydrate
Bagel with:				
2 Tbsp cream cheese	262	39%	12%	49%
2 Tbsp Smucker's Low-Sugar Spread	211	6%	11%	83%
English Muffin with:				
1 Tbsp margerine	237	47%	8%	45%
1 Tbsp Smucker's Low-Sugar Spread	159	6%	11%	83%

Sufficiently impressed? I have just one more argument for low- or no-sugar preserves. The calorie difference (which in the land of preserves usually also means the sugar difference) between regular jams and jellies and the "no sugar added" (juice sweetened) types is worth mentioning.

- Regular jams, jellies, and preserves, 1 tablespoon = 55 calories
- Smucker's Low-Sugar Boysenberry Spread, 1 tablespoon = 24 calories
- Fruit juice sweetened brands, 1 tablespoon = 6 calories (averages)

If you use a couple tablespoons of preserves every day on your toast, this adds up to a savings of around 700 calories a week if you choose fruit juice sweetened preserves versus full-strength sugar types. (And you can bet those are 700 refined sugar calories you're saving yourself from.)

Soups Can Be Good Food

Soup. So delicious, especially on a cold winter day, yet quite a project to make from scratch. The way I see it, we have a couple options. Buy canned or packaged soups, but only those low in fat and not too terribly high in sodium, or make a big pot of soup, freezing several containers full for future quick and warm meals.

The key to low-fat soups, whether homemade or from a can, is to choose the clear broth types most of the time and leave the creamy and cheesy types for those special occasions. Campbell's Creamy Chicken Mushroom Soup & Sauce has 60 percent of its calories from fat. Campbell's Cheddar Cheese Soup has 55 percent of calories from fat. See what I mean? Campbell's Zesty Tomato, on the other hand, has 10 percent of its calories from fat, while Campbell's Home Cookin' Country Vegetable has 15 percent.

Now, sodium, that's another story. Sodium doesn't discriminate between the clear and the creamy soup types. High amounts can be found in both. Campbell's has a "Special Request" line out on the shelves with one-third less salt. Even these selections have around 500 milligrams of sodium per 1-cup serving. Look at enough cans and packages of soup and you can even see numbers in the low one-thousands.

After paying the soup aisle a little visit, I was amazed at the vast assortment of varieties lining shelf after shelf, in cans where you add water or milk, in single-serving envelopes or plastic tubs, now even in 10 3/4-ounce ready-to-serve cans. Soup isn't just the chicken noodle variety of yester-year. Today, soup is Lipton's Minestrone (9 percent calories from fat) or Lemon Chicken from Lipton's "Lite" line (less than 20 percent of calories from fat).

Before I leave the subject of soup for the duration of the book, I'll share with you the "something new" I learned the other day while walking through the soup section. If you add 4 ounces of skim milk instead of whole milk to 4 ounces of condensed Campbell's Creamy Natural Broccoli Soup, it transforms into a 26 percent calories-from-fat soup.

Let's take a look at the better soups I found in my supermarket that had less than 25 percent of calories from fat.

Low-fat Soups

Per 8-ounce prepared serving, unless noted

Brand	Calories	Fat (gm)	% Calories from Fat	Sodium (mg)
Tomato Based:				
Campbell's Ready to Serve Healthy Request				
Hearty Minestrone	90	2	20%	420
Healthy Choice Ready to Serve (per 7.5-oz. serving)				
Tomato Garden	130	3	21%	510
Minestrone	160	1	6%	520
Campbell's Condensed Soup				
Tomato Soup	90	2	20%	670
Progresso Healthy Classics (per 9.5-oz. serving)				
Tomato	90	2	20%	1120
Hearty Minestrone	90	2	20%	760
Minestrone	120	3	22.5%	910
Broth Based:				
Progresso Healthy Classics (9.5-oz. servings)				
Chicken Rice	80	2	22.5%	440
Chicken & Wild Rice	120	3	22.5%	850

Brand	Calories	Fat (gm)	% Calories from Fat	Sodium (mg)
Vegetable	90	1	10%	810
Chicken Noodle	90	2	20%	870
Chicken Barley	110	3	24.5%	790
Chicken Rice with Vegetables	120	3	22.5%	800
Tortellini in Chicken Broth	80	2	22.5%	870
Campbell's Ready to Serve Healthy Request				
Hearty Chicken Noodle	120	2	15%	460
Hearty Chicken Vegetable	80	2	22.5%	470
Hearty Chicken Rice	110	3	24.5%	480
Hearty Vegetable Beef	120	2	15%	460
Vegetable	90	1	10%	480
Campbell's Condensed Healthy Request Soups				
Vegetable Beef	90	2	20%	500
Chicken Rice	60	2	30%	480
Chicken Noodle	60	2	30%	460
Healthy Choice Ready to Serve (per 7.5 oz. serving)				
Turkey Vegetable	110	3	25%	540
Chicken Pasta	100	2	18%	560
Garden Vegetable	100	1	9%	560
Country Vegetable	120	1	8%	540
Chicken Rice	90	1	10%	510
Chicken Noodle	90	2	20%	540
Beef and Potato	110	1	8%	550
Vegetable Beef	130	1	7%	530

Bean Soups:

Brand	Calories	Fat (gm)	% Calories from Fat	Sodium (mg)
Healthy Choice Ready to Serve				
Split Pea and Ham	170	3	16%	460
Bean and Ham	220	4	16%	480
Lentil	140	1	6%	480
Campbell's Condensed Soup				
Split Pea	160	4	22.5%	780
Progresso Healthy Classics (per 9.5 oz. serving)				
Hearty Black Bean	140	2	13%	820
Lentil	130	2	14%	840

Brand	Calories	Fat (gm)	% Calories from Fat	Sodium (mg)
Creamy (prepared with skim milk unless otherwise noted):				
Campbell's Ready to Serve Healthy Request				
Calm Chowder	100	3	27%	490
Campbell's Condensed Healthy Request				
Cream of Broccoli	100	2	18%	440
Cream of Mushroom (prepared with water)	60	2	30%	480
Cream of Celery	100	2	18%	480
Cream of Chicken	70	2	26%	490
Campbell's Condensed Soup				
Clam Chowder (prepared with 2% milk)	130	4	26%	940

Bottled Sauces

I keep a bottle of spaghetti sauce in my refrigerator at all times. (I won't leave the supermarket without it.) In a pinch, it can substitute for pizza sauce, sauce for a quick quesadilla, pasta sauce (add non- or low-fat milk for a creamy variation), or topping for a 5-minute microwave potato—along with part-skim cheese, of course.

But the lesson here is to stock up only on spaghetti sauces that are themselves low in fat. That way if you add them to low-fat foods (pasta noodles, potatoes, rice, corn tortillas), you are sure to produce a low-fat meal. And here they are:

Bottled Sauces

Per 1/2 cup (4 oz.)

Brand	Calories	% Calories from Fat	Fat	Sodium (mg)
Enrico's				
Ragu Fino Italian (most varieties)	80-90	34% - 30%	3	490
Ragu Thick & Hearty (most varieties)	100	27%	3	460

Brand	Calories	% Calories from Fat	Fat	Sodium (mg)
Today's Recipe				
Chunky Mushroom	50	185	1	370
Garlic & Herbs	50	18%	1	370
Healthy Choice				
Chunky Mushroom	45	0	0	350
Traditional	40	<22.5%	<1	350
Garlic & Onion	40	0	0	350
Italian Chunky Vegetable	40	0	0	350
Garlic & Herbs	40	22.5%	<1	350
Campbell's Healthy Request				
Fresh mushroom (traditional)	50	0	0	360
Classico				
Tomato Basil	60	45%	3	340
Mushroom & Ripe Olives	50	36%	2	470
Spicy Red Pepper	50	36%	2	250
Prego				
Tomato Basil	100	185	2	370
Mushroom & Diced Tomato	100	27%	3	480
Garden Combination	80	22.5%	2	420
Mushroom with Extra Spice	100	27%	3	450
Mushroom & Green Pepper	90	30%	3	410

Undressing Your Salad

You're staring down at an innocent bed of salad greens, thinking to yourself, "Boy, this must be good for me! Look at all those cucumber slices, tomato wedges, red cabbage strips." Meanwhile you're tipping a bottle of creamy dressing over and around your salad bowl, ruining its healthful effect. Are salads healthful? Let's take a closer look at a generic bowl of salad—and especially at that bottle of salad dressing.

Your basic 2 cups of shredded romaine lettuce topped with 1/4 of a medium cucumber, 1 medium tomato, and 1/4 cup of shredded red cabbage is indeed a low-calorie, low-fat, low-sodium dish—at least until you dress it. It has a total of 70 calories, 10 percent of them from fat, and a grand total of 25 milligrams of sodium. Pretty impressive? But what does the typical American do to this garden-fresh masterpiece?

If you use regular salad dressings, even a little bit, it is almost impossible to keep the percent of calories from fat in your salad decent. The calories will start to pour out real quick, too. Salad dressings typically have 70 to 100 calories per tablespoon. Some people pour about 1/4 cup (4 tablespoons!) to 1/2 cup (8 tablespoons!) onto their once low-fat and low-calorie lettuce and vegetables.

This means if you add 1/4 cup of dressing, your salad has just become a 350-calorie dish, with 85 percent of those calories from FAT! And the ante for sodium has just been upped to around 475 milligrams.

So what's a health-conscious, salad-loving person to do? First of all, trade in your measuring cup for a tablespoon measure, and try to keep your pouring down to 2 tablespoons. Then, start sampling some of the lower calorie (thus lower fat) dressing alternatives. These days "reduced calorie" salad dressings come in all types of brands and flavors. Those salad dressings lower in anything worth mentioning are listed here. Unfortunately, it seems that no one offers reduced sodium in a salad dressing—at least not yet. The sodium is up there (they're all over 100 milligrams per tablespoon) so don't even think about grabbing that salt shaker.

The following items contain no more than 2 grams of fat and no more than 300 milligrams sodium per 1-ounce (2 tablespoons) serving.

Seven Seas Free–Ranch

Healthy Sensations Fat Free–Honey Dijon, Ranch, Italian, Chunky Bleu Cheese, Thousand Island

Wish Bone Lite–Russian

Walden Farms Fat Free–French, Thousand Island, Creamy Italian

Kraft Free–Bleu Cheese, Catalina, Italian, Ranch, Thousand Island

Hidden Valley Ranch Low Fat–Italian Parmesan, Honey Dijon Ranch, Original Ranch, French, Bleu Cheese

Bernstein's Light Fantastic–Classico Italian, Creamy Dijon, Creamy Dill, Oriental

Some of these salad dressings make great low-fat pasta vinaigrettes and meat or vegetable marinades!

So, say you're now pouring 2 tablespoons of Bernstein's Italian with Cheese (low calorie) dressing over your generic salad. Your salad now contains about 82 calories and a little more than 10 percent of calories from fat.

Sounds a little better, doesn't it? Hopefully something we can all live with, because if not, we'll have to start calling salad a dessert!

Make Way for the Mayo

One of the supermarket sections that has undergone a face lift lately is the mayonnaise shelf. My advice as a nutritionist used to be quite simple: "Hold the mayo." Now things are a little more complicated. Many varieties of reduced calorie (which also means reduced fat) mayonnaise are now available on most supermarket shelves.

Regular mayonnaise has an average of 98 calories per tablespoon. (Think of that when you're dipping into the gallon-sized jug of mayonnaise.) And that mayo has 11 grams of fat! For the mayonnaise look-alikes to have half the fat, they should have 5 or fewer grams of fat per tablespoon. Well, guess what! Several of them do! Here they are:

Reduced-Fat Mayonnaise

Per Tablespoon

Brand	Calories	Fat (gms)	Cholesterol (mgs)	Sodium (mgs)
Weight Watchers Light	50	5	5	100
Smart Beat	40	4	0	110
Best Foods Light	50	5	5	115
Best Foods Reduced Fat	40	3	0	160
Kraft Light	60	5	0	110
Kraft Free	8	0	0	125
Miracle Whip Free	15	0	0	105
Miracle Whip Light	40	3	0	120

What about the "cholesterol-free" types versus the others? Well, as you can see from the list, once the fat has been cut down to size (making it reduced calorie), the cholesterol also goes way down. The ones above WITH cholesterol only have around 5 measly milligrams per tablespoon. So I say, go with the one you like best . . . the one that will tempt you away from using regular fatty mayonnaise the most (as long as it's lower in fat)—for me, this is Best Foods Reduced Fat Mayo.

Chapter 4

Big Mac Attack: Cutting the Fat at the Top Fast Food Chains

So there you sit, in the middle of nowhere. Your stomach has growled at least three times, so you get off at the next exit where you recognize a fast food chain. You already thought about, visualized, and salivated over what to order. That's one of the best things about fast food chains—reliability. You know what to expect whether you're in L.A., London, or Nebraska. You never quite know with the "Dick's Diner" or the "Alice's Grill" types—except if their parking lot is empty, you know to stay away!

Or say you're running errands on your lunch hour, with 15 minutes to grab something to eat on your way back to the office. Where else can you get a meal in minutes? (If there's a drive-through window, you don't even have to leave your car if you don't want to.) That's the other great thing about fast food—it really is fast!

But I don't have to remind you about the advantages of fast food. America obviously already has them down pat. The problems start when it comes to ordering.

Five Rules for Feeding in the Fast Lane

Rule #1. Learn to Limit Total Fat

Start off by ordering a sandwich or entree with close to or less than 35 percent of calories from fat. Then, when you order other items with much less fat, you can be sure the total fast food meal will be under 30 percent of calories from fat. The best and the worst from each of a variety of fast food chains is listed below:

Fast Food Choices

Arby's–

Best Bets

	Calories	% Calories from fat	Fat (grams)	Sodium (mg.)
Cinnamon Nut Danish	360	27.5%	11	105
Blueberry Muffin	240	26%	7	200
Arby Q Roast Beef	389	35%	15	1268
Grilled Chicken Barbeque	386	30.5%	13	1002
Plain Baked Potato	240	7.5%	2	58
Roast Chicken Salad	204	32%	7	508
Light Roast Beef Deluxe	294	31%	10	826
Light Roast Turkey Deluxe	260	21%	6	1262
Light Roast Chicken Deluxe	276	23%	7	777
Old Fashioned Chicken Noodle Soup	99	16%	1.8	929

Worst Bets

	Calories	% Calories from fat	Fat (grams)	Sodium (mg.)
Toastix	420	53%	25	440
Bacon Biscuit	318	51%	18	904
Sausage Biscuit	460	62%	32	1000
Plain Croissant	260	54%	15.6	300
Bacon/Egg Croissant	430	63%	30	720
Ham/Cheese Croissant	345	54%	21	939

	Calories	% Calories from fat	Fat (grams)	Sodium (mg.)
Mushroom/Cheese Croissant	493	69%	38	935
Sausage/Egg Croissant	519	68%	39	632
Sausage Platter	640	58%	41	861
Bacon Platter	593	50%	33	880
Bac 'N Cheddar Deluxe	512	55%	31.5	1094
Italian Sub	671	52%	39	2062
Tuna Sub	663	50%	37	1342
Potato Cakes	204	53%	12	397
Deluxe Baked Potato	621	53%	36	605
Wisconsin Cheese Soup	281	58%	18	1084

Burger King—

Best Bets

	Calories	% Calories from fat	Fat (grams)	Sodium (mg.)
Hamburger	260	35%	10	500
BK Broiler chicken	280	32%	10	770
Chunky Chicken salad w/ light Italian dressing	172	26%	5	1153

Worst Bets

	Calories	% Calories from fat	Fat (grams)	Sodium (mg.)
Whopper with cheese	660	52%	38	1190
Double Whopper	800	54%	48	940
Double Whopper with cheese	890	56%	55	1250
Bacon Double Cheeseburger	470	54%	28	800
Bacon Double Cheeseburger deluxe	530	56%	33	860
Double Cheeseburger	450	50%	25	840
Ocean Catch Fish	450	56%	28	760
Chicken Tenders, 6 pieces	236	50%	13	541
Onion Rings	339	50%	19	628
Croissan'wich with bacon, egg and cheese	353	59%	23	780
Croissan'wich with sausage, egg and cheese	534	67%	40	985
Croissan'wich with ham, egg and cheese	351	56%	22	1373

	Calories	% Calories from fat	Fat (grams)	Sodium (mg.)
Breakfast buddy with sausage, egg and cheese	255	56%	16	492
French Toast sticks	440	55%	27	490
Hashbrowns	213	51%	12	318

Carl's Jr–

Best Bets

	Calories	% Calories from fat	Fat (grams)	Sodium (mg.)
Charbroiler BBQ Chicken sandwich	310	17%	6	680
Teriyaki Chicken	330	16%	6	830
Santa Fe Chicken	540	22%	13	1180
Lite Potato	290	3%	1	60
English muffin with margarine	190	24%	5	280
Blueberry Muffin	340	24%	9	300
Bran Muffin	310	20%	7	370

Worst Bets

	Calories	% Calories from fat	Fat (grams)	Sodium (mg.)
Famous Star Hamburger	610	56%	38	890
Super Star	820	58%	53	1210
Double Western Bacon Cheeseburger	1030	55%	63	1810
Bacon & Cheese Potato	730	53%	43	1670
Breakfast Burrito	430	54%	26	740
Scrambled Eggs	120	67.5%	9	105
Sausage, 1 patty	190	85%	18	520
Bacon, 2 strips	45	80%	4	150
Hash Brown Nuggets	270	57%	17	410
Zucchini (fried)	390	53%	23	1040
Crisscut Fries, reg.	330	60%	22	890
Chicken Strips, 6 pieces	260	66%	19	600

Hardee's–

Best Bets

	Calories	% Calories from fat	Fat (grams)	Sodium (mg.)
Three Pancakes	280	6%	2	890
Three Pancakes with 1 Sausage Pattie	430	33%	16	1290
Three Pancakes with 2 Bacon Strips	350	23%	9	1110
Hamburger	260	35%	10	510
Regular Roast Beef	280	35%	11	870
Hot Ham 'N Cheese	330	33%	12	1420
Turkey Sub	390	16%	7	1420
Roast Beef Sub	370	12%	5	1400
Ham Sub	370	17%	7	1400
Combo Sub	380	14%	6	1440
Chicken Fillet	370	32%	13	1060
Grilled Chicken Breast	310	26%	9	890
Mashed Potatoes (4 oz.) with gravy (1.5 oz.)	90	<14%	<2	520

Worst Bets

	Calories	% Calories from fat	Fat (grams)	Sodium (mg.)
Rise 'N Shine Biscuit	320	51%	18	740
Sausage Biscuit	440	57%	28	1100
Sausage & Egg Biscuit	490	57%	31	1150
Bacon Biscuit	360	52.5%	21	950
Bacon & Egg Biscuit	410	53%	24	990
Bacon, Egg & Cheese Biscuit	460	55%	28	1220
Canadian Rise 'N Shine Biscuit	470	52%	27	1550
Steak Biscuit	500	52%	29	1320
Steak & Egg Biscuit	550	52%	32	1370
Big Country Breakfast (sausage)	850	60%	57	1980
Big Country Breakfast (bacon)	660	54.5%	40	1540
Big Country Breakfast (country ham)	670	51%	38	2870
Hash Rounds	230	55%	14	560
Quarter-Pound Cheeseburger	500	52%	29	1060
Big Deluxe Burger	500	53%	30	760
Bacon Cheeseburger	610	57.5%	39	1030

	Calories	% Calories from fat	Fat (grams)	Sodium (mg.)
Mushroom 'N Swiss Burger	490	50%	27	940
Big Twin	450	50%	25	580
Hot Dog	290	50%	16	760
Fried Chicken Breast	340	50%	19	659
Fried Chicken Wing	205	57%	13	274
Fried Chicken Thigh	370	63%	26	489
Coleslaw (4 oz.)	240	75%	20	340

Jack in the Box–

Best Bets

	Calories	% Calories from fat	Fat (grams)	Sodium (mg.)
Beef Teriyaki Bowl	740	7%	6	1420
Chicken Teriyaki Bowl	720	3%	2.5	1460
Pancake Platter	612	32%	22	888
Chicken Fajita Pita	292	25%	8	703
Sesame Breadsticks	70	26%	2	110

Worst Bets

	Calories	% Calories from fat	Fat (grams)	Sodium (mg.)
The Colossus	1095	62%	75	1340
Sharp Cheddar Cheeseburger	859	58%	55	1104
Sausage Crescent	584	66%	43	1012
Scrambled Egg Platter	559	52%	32	1060
Supreme Crescent	547	67%	40	1053
Hash Browns	156	63%	11	312
Double Cheeseburger	467	52%	27	842
Jumbo Jack	584	52%	34	733
Jumbo Jack with Cheese	677	53%	40	1090
Bacon Bacon Cheeseburger	705	57%	45	1240
Grilled Sourdough Burger	712	63%	50	1140
Ultimate Cheeseburger	942	66%	69	1176
Chicken Supreme	641	55%	39	1470
Country Fried Steak Sandwich	450	50%	25	891
Taco Salad (includes salsa)	503	55%	31	1600
Super Taco	281	54%	17	718
Seasoned Curly Fries	358	50%	20	1030
Onion Rings	380	54%	23	451

Kentucky Fried Chicken–

Best Bets

	Calories	% Calories from fat	Fat (grams)	Sodium (mg.)
Mashed Potatoes & Gravy	71	25%	2	339
Corn on-the-cob	90	20%	2	11

Worst Bets

	Calories	% Calories from fat	Fat (grams)	Sodium (mg.)
Chicken Littles	169	53%	10	331
Crispy Fries	294	52%	17	761
Colonel's Chicken	482	50%	27	1060
Hot Wings (6)	471	63%	33	1230

* All the fried chicken selections contain more than 50% calories from fat, except the Skinfree Crispy Center Breast and Drumstick which have 49% calories from fat (16 and 9 grams of fat, respectively). Listed below is the nutrition information for the side and center breasts only (which, of all the chicken selections are the lowest in % calories from fat.)

	Calories	% Calories from fat	Fat (grams)	Sodium (mg.)
Skinfree Crispy:				
side breast	293	52%	17	410
Original Recipe:				
side breast	245	55%	15	604
center breast	260	66%	14	609
Extra Tasty Crispy:				
side breast	379	64%	27	646
center breast	344	55%	21	636
Hot & Spicy:				
side breast	398	61%	27	922
center breast	382	59%	25	905

Long John Silver's–

Best Bets

	Calories	% Calories from fat	Fat (grams)	Sodium (mg.)
Fish w/ lemon crumb, rice, green beans, slaw, roll, no margarine	570	19%	12	1470
Light Portion Fish w/lemon crumb 2-pc.with rice and small salad (no dressing)	290	15.5%	5	690
Chicken (includes rice, green beans, slaw and roll, no margarine)	550	24.5%	15	1670
3-pc. Fish, lemon crumb	150	6%	1	370
Chicken-Light Herb	120	30%	4	570
Batter-dipped fish sandwich, no sauce	340	34%	13	890
Batter-dipped chicken sandwich, no sauce	280	26%	8	790
Ocean Chef Salad without dressing	110	8%	1	730
Hushpuppies, 1 piece	70	26%	2	25
Rice	160	17%	3	340
Roll	110	8%	<1	170

Worst Bets

	Calories	% Calories from fat	Fat (grams)	Sodium (mg.)
Fish & Fries, 2 pieces	610	55%	37	1480
Shrimp, 10 pieces, with 2 hushpuppies, fries and slaw	840	50%	47	1630
1 Fish, 1 Chicken & fries	550	52%	32	1380
Fish & Shrimp (2 fish, 8 shrimp, 2 hushpuppies, fries & slaw)	1140	51%	65	2440
Fish, Shrimp & Chicken (2 fish, 5 shrimp, 1 chicken, fries, slaw and 2 hushpuppies	1160	50%	65	2590
Fish, Shrimp & Clams (2 fish, 4 shrimp, 3-oz clams, fries, slaw and 2 hushpuppies	1240	51%	70	2630
Seafood Salad without dressing	380	73%	31	980
Batter-dipped fish, 1 piece	180	55%	11	490
Batter-dipped shrimp, 1 piece	30	60%	2	80
Seafood Gumbo w/cod	120	60%	8	740
Fries, 1 order	250	54%	15	500
Corn Cobbette, 1 piece	140	51%	8	0

McDonald's–

Best Bets

	Calories	% Calories from fat	Fat (grams)	Sodium (mg.)
Hamburger	255	32%	9	490
McLean Burger	255	32%	9	490
Chunky Chicken Salad with Lite Vinaigrette	98	27%	6	470
Egg McMuffin	280	35%	11	710
English Muffin w/ Spread	170	21%	4	285
Hotcakes w/ Margarine & Syrup	440	24.5%	12	685
Cheerios	80	11%	1	210
Wheaties	90	10%	1	220
Fat-Free Apple Bran Muffin	180	0%	0	200
Vanilla Lowfat Frozen Yogurt Cone	105	9%	1	80
Filet-O-Fish without tartar sauce	290	34%	11	580
McChicken no mayonnaise	343	31%	12	655

Worst Bets

	Calories	% Calories from fat	Fat (grams)	Sodium (mg.)
Chicken McNuggets, 6 pieces	270	50%	15	580
Sausage McMuffin	345	52%	20	710
Sausage McMuffin with Egg	430	52%	25	920
Biscuit w/ sausage	420	60%	28	1040
Biscuit w/ Sausage & Egg	505	59%	33	1210
Biscuit w/ Bacon, Egg & Cheese	440	53%	26	1215
Sausage	160	84%	15	310
Scrambled Eggs (2)	140	64%	10	290
Breakfast Burrito	280	55%	17	580

Taco Bell–

Best Bets

	Calories	% Calories from fat	Fat (grams)	Sodium (mg.)
Bean Burrito	387	32.5%	14	1148
Chicken Burrito	334	32%	12	880
Combo Burrito	407	35%	16	1136

Worst Bets

	Calories	% Calories from fat	Fat (grams)	Sodium (mg.)
Taco	183	54%	11	276
Soft Taco Supreme	272	53%	16	554
Taco Supreme	230	59%	15	276
Nachos Supreme	367	66%	27	471
Beef MexiMelt	266	51%	15	689
Chicken MexiMelt	257	52%	15	779
Mexican Pizza	575	58%	37	1031
Taco Salad	905	61%	61	910
Taco Salad w/o shell	484	58%	31	680

Wendy's–

Best Bets

	Calories	% Calories from fat	Fat (grams)	Sodium (mg.)
Plain Baked Potato	300	<3%	<1	20
Bacon & Cheese Potato	510	30%	17	1170
Broccoli & Cheese Potato	450	28%	14	450
Sour Cream & Chives Potato	370	15%	6	35
Small Chili	190	28%	6	670
Jr. Hamburger	270	30%	9	590
Grilled Chicken sandwich	290	22%	7	670
Breaded Chicken no mayonnaise	380	31%	13	695

Worst Bets

	Calories	% Calories from fat	Fat (grams)	Sodium (mg.)
Chicken Nuggets, 6 pieces	280	64%	20	600
Jr. Bacon Cheeseburger	440	51%	25	870
Country Fried Steak	460	51%	26	880

Exceptions to Rule #1: How to Dilute Total Fat

A friend of mine, after hearing about my fast food rules, said, "Just tell me what I need to order so I don't have to give up my French fries." My sister had a similar reaction. "You might succeed in getting me off the quarter pounder with cheese and onto the little hamburgers, but I'm not ordering the plain hamburgers—no matter how much healthier they are."

I realize we all have our fast food obsessions (although I'm never telling what mine is.) It's important to take them into account. After all, if you set unrealistic goals for yourself, you'll never be able to stick with the program. Maybe you've even found the loophole in Rule #1. If not, I'll let you in on it.

The bottom line to Rule #1 is to make sure your total fast food meal is less than 30 percent of calories from fat. Theoretically, you could order a sandwich or side order that was somewhere in the 40 percent range, adding the necessary carbo calories, such as orange juice or salad with vegetables (with low-calorie dressing, of course), bringing the percent of calories from fat for the meal down to an acceptable level.

So let's try to solve the "gotta have the French fries" or "cheese on the burger" blues.

The French Fry Obsession:

1. Start by placing Carl's Jr. French fries (for example) at the top of your list.

    French fries = 360 calories (42 percent from fat), or 17 grams of fat

    Remember: You can calculate grams of fat from the percent of calories from fat by first multiplying the calories per serving by the percent of calories from fat, divided by 100.

    Then divide this number by 9 (the number of calories in each gram of fat).

2. Add on the lower fat sandwiches or side orders, such as Carl's Charbroiler Chicken sandwich, with 320 calories, 14 percent of them from fat, and 5 grams of fat.

I calculated this by multiplying 320 calories by 14 (percent of calories from fat) divided by 100. Then I divided this number by 9. My answer is 5 grams of fat.

3. Let's see how much orange juice you need to drink to get down to 30 percent of total calories from fat:

Each small glass of orange juice at Carl's has 94 calories and 1 gram of fat.

If you can manage to guzzle just one small orange juice with your fries and sandwich, for a total of 774 calories, you'll have brought the percentage of fat calories down to 27%. So the fries will work—provided you're not on a weight reduction plan that limits calories as well as fat.

The Cheese on the Burger Obsession

1. Start with your cheeseburger from McDonald's at 318 calories, with 45 percent of those calories from fat and 16 grams of fat.

2. Add some carbohydrate calories, such as a sack of carrot sticks. (You probably have to bring these from home.)

3. Buy 2 grapefruit juice containers, each with 6 ounces and 80 calories, with no grams of fat, or some orange juice. Viola! You've got your cheese on the burger and a fairly healthful meal to boot, with 518 total calories, 28 percent of which are from fat.

Rule #2. Zip-Lock Carbohydrates

Have you heard of the game "Find the missing complex carbohydrates?" (This is very popular in nutrition circles.) I'll give you a hint. With fast food this usually refers to fruits and vegetables. The purpose of the game isn't just to find them but to then plan them into your fast food meal.

If you're lucky, some chains sell orange juice or let you make your own vegetable-packed salad. If not, you should plan to bring your own. "Bring vegetables and fruits with me?" you ask. I know this might take some getting used to. Your co-workers might laugh a little—maybe a lot—when you pull your zip-lock bag filled with broccoli or carrot sticks and your apple or orange out of your briefcase or purse. But you'll probably only have to explain the first time. Maybe they'll even start to tote their carbohydrates with them, too.

Practice Scenario #1:

You've decided to go to Wendy's for lunch. You're going to order the chicken breast sandwich and go to the salad bar, adding only 2 tablespoons of reduced-calorie dressing. (By the way, you're going to have to carry a measuring spoon with you, because what you think is a tablespoon and what it really is can be two very different animals.) In this case, only your fruit carbohydrate is missing. You can either order an orange juice or bring some fruit with you. Buy a bottle of juice or a piece of fruit at the market on the way, or bring it from home.

Practice Scenario #2:

There you sit in 5 o'clock traffic. You're tired, frustrated, and worst of all, starving to the point of food fantasizing. Just then you spot a yellow Taco Bell in the distance.

You decide to order the combo burrito. Okay, so let's go through nutrition roll call: The tortilla definitely counts as the bread/starch group; it might be pushing it a bit, but you could consider the chopped tomatoes as part of your fruit serving (tomatoes really are fruit). But where's the vegetable? Looks like some carrot sticks are in order.

Rule #3. Dress Your Food Yourself

You may need to come equipped with some toppings. If the fast food chain you patronize doesn't offer a low-calorie salad dressing, you still have these options:

- You can measure a couple of tablespoons of your low-calorie dressing from home into a small container and bring it with you.
- If you typically munch your fast food meal back at work, you can bring a bottle of low-cal dressing to the office and keep it in the refrigerator for a fat-reducing salad.

How to Avoid Those Slabs of Butter

If you order a plain baked potato, you can add your own non- or low-fat yogurt or grated part-skim mozzarella cheese.

- Buy a small container of yogurt on the way to the fast food place.
- Bring yogurt or cheese from home, keeping it in the refrigerator at work.

Rule #4. Beware of Fast Food Liquids!

I know, I know, it's convenient and tempting to order your drink there. But fast food chains typically don't sell you a drink free from fat, sugar, or artificial sweeteners.

Nonfat milk, mineral water, and juices, as well as fruits and vegetables (and I'm not talking about the slice of tomato or leaf of lettuce on your hamburger) are simply not the common fare at fast food chains, at least not yet. So be ready to make a pit stop for them on the way or bring them from home.

Rule #5. Once is Enough.

Eat fast food a maximum of once a day. Most fast food items are loaded with sodium, and if you're trying to stay within the health guidelines (less than 4 grams of sodium per day), two large fast food meals might push you way over the edge.

Before you even start your work day, you could be half way to your sodium limit. A Croissan'wich with ham, egg, and cheese at Burger King totals 1,373 milligrams of sodium. Now on to lunch—an Arby's Italian Sub Sandwich by itself has 2,062 milligrams of sodium. Or a Tuna Sub totals 1,342 milligrams of sodium.

Needless to say, don't even think about salting your fast food at the table. Leave those salt packets alone. Believe me, the salt's already in there.

Other Tips for Fast Lane Food

1. *Cut the cream.* Wipe off the mayonnaise or tartar sauce (all the creamy type sauces) on your sandwiches, or order them "your way" without sauces. Just try spreading a little catsup or mustard instead. It makes a BIG difference—fat and calorie-wise.

   Fast food companies supposedly test and retest their recipes based on what the average consumer wants. It's hard for me to believe the average American really wants two tablespoons of gloppy tartar sauce on a Fillet-O-Fish sandwich. Evidently McDonald's does. Or that a BK Broiler chicken sandwich "needs" two tablespoons of mayonnaise. Still that's how much Burger King squirts on.

2. *Double your pleasure, double your fat.* Avoid the "deluxe" or "double" this or that type of burgers and you'll rescue yourself from a whopping amount of fat and calories. Here are some examples:

   • Jack in the Box Ultimate Cheeseburger, 942 calories, 66 percent from fat

   • McDonald's Big Mac, 750 calories, 55 percent from fat

   • Carl's Jr. Double Western Bacon Cheeseburger, 890 calories, 54 percent from fat

3. *Fatty fryers.* Avoid the fried chicken and chicken pieces. Are those six itsy bitsy bite-size nuggets really worth 323 calories, especially when 56 percent of those calories are from fat? And that's before dipping them.

4. *Pizza to go, hold the fat.* When ordering pizza, stick with ordering vegetables on top. Skipping the pepperoni, salami, or sausage will save you from many extra calories and much fat.

Salad Bar Minefield

When in the salad bar, remember to keep your distance from cheese, chow mein noodles, coleslaw, croutons, eggs, pasta salad, and mayonnaise-loaded salads, such as macaroni and egg. Instead, load up on the greens, raw vegetables, and beans and use the low-calorie dressings or bring them from home.

Blowing the Whistle on Some Fast Food Frauds

To Eat or Not to Eat the Shell?

Taco Bell has a taco salad that comes in a deep fried (very attractive) flour tortilla shell. And everyone who orders it, I am sure, ponders whether or not to crunch the shell into bite-size pieces and mix it into the salad, bite off chunks, or toss it, quickly, into the nearest trash can. Well, ponder no more. They must really be deep frying those babies extra long—each has about 400 calories, with 67 percent from fat. That's a high price to pay for "cute."

Does Kentucky Really "Do Chicken Right?"

Only if you like GREASE! What does the Colonel "do" to a normally low-fat chicken breast? An Original Recipe chicken breast is 270 calories, 48 to 52 percent from fat. Extra Crispy, which is really extra fatty, is 354 calories, with 53 to 60 percent from fat. For comparison sake (or shock value), a regular unadulterated broiled chicken breast (without the skin) is 140 calories, 21 percent from fat.

The Criminal—Mr. Mayo

It's bad enough that fast food chicken and fish patties are deep fried in grease, but squirting mayonnaise or tartar sauce (Mr. Mayo's daughter) on top is absolutely criminal. Take Burger King's Chicken Specialty Sandwich (which comes with a chicken patty, bun, mayonnaise, and lettuce) with a total of 688 calories, 52 percent of them from fat. Scrape off the mayo—or order it "your way" without the mayo—and suddenly we're talking about a 495-calorie sandwich, with only 36 percent of calories from fat. That's good enough to qualify for a "Best Bet."

Big Mac (Heart) Attack

Bite into a Big Mac and you bite into some big calories—and fat calories at that. One Big Mac has 570 calories, 55 percent from fat, along with 980 milligrams of sodium.

What is it about the Big Mac that makes it such a fat snack? Could it be the slices of processed cheese? Or the heaping tablespoons of thousand island-like dressing? (Of course they call it their "special sauce.") Or maybe it's the two hamburger patties with only the three slices of bun?

If you find the "stacked-up" look attractive in the Big Mac, why don't you order two regular (little) hamburgers and place one on top of the other before eating.

Chapter

Five Star Dining

Eating Out is America's favorite pastime. Often, even when we're "eating in," we're really "eating out" by buying take-out food to eat at home. I don't know about you, but when I'm dining in a restaurant my mind automatically snaps into its "splurge" mode. This may be because when I was growing up, eating out, even at McDonald's, was usually a special occasion.

Don't get me wrong. I'm not against the occasional "what the heck, this time I'm going to order what I really want, and then I'm going to order dessert" approach. But with eating out becoming a daily ritual for some of us, this splurging stuff can get way out of hand. So to help you (and me) out of this splurge rut, I put together some tips to help us keep FAT calories in line when eating out, except for those rare and truly "bonus" occasions.

The Before-Dinner Ditties

The bread sitting pretty in that basket on the table is usually fine. It's the clumps of chilled butter that can get you into some major calories from fat before dinner is even served. One slice of French bread has 70 calories, about 10 percent from fat. A small pat of butter (1 teaspoon) has 36 calories—all of them from fat. Put them together and what have you got? A fairly fatty appetizer. If buttering your bread is nonnegotiable, then try to keep the butter to a half teaspoon per slice, which totals around 88 calories with the slice of bread, with 31 percent of calories from fat, or less.

When it comes to soups, order the clear, broth-type soups, such as chicken noodle, bean, beef-vegetable, or tomato-based instead of the creamy-type soups. (One exception is the clear broth-like French onion soup, which has only 100 calories per cup, but is 70 percent fat calories). For example, beef barley soup has about 195 calories per cup, with 6 percent of calories from fat. Cream of cauliflower soup, on the other hand, has 280 calories and is 71 percent calories from fat.

And you usually can't get into too much trouble with a shrimp or crab cocktail. Half a cup has about 65 calories (10 percent from fat) and a tablespoon of cocktail sauce only adds about 15 calories.

Then there's always the raw vegetable platters, which can be a fresh, crisp, and low-fat way to work in your daily dose of vegetables, as long as you make sure the creamy dip is on the side and that you really do "dip" and not "scoop." Better yet, use a small spoon to scoop out about half a tablespoon onto your plate and use only that amount to dress your veggies.

To help you stay on the right course when eating out, follow the tips below.

1. Watch out for anything described as "creamy," "breaded," or "fried." Also watch for anything dressed with mayonnaise. (Remember mayo is made from egg yolks and oil.) It's wise to beware of coleslaw, potato, or macaroni salads.

2. Avoid ordering meat, poultry, or seafood portions larger than about 4 ounces cooked (6 ounces raw) or take the excess home for tomorrow's sandwich.

3. Order your meat, poultry, or seafood grilled or broiled (without added butter or fats) or poached.

4. If your entree is ordinarily "sautéed" or "simmered" in cream or butter, ask that it be simmered in wine instead.

5. Most sauces and dressings can quickly get you into fat calories *big time*. So, order them on the side so you know how much you're adding. If, for example, you want some melted butter with your steamed clams or prawns but you want to keep the meal low in fat, take your small spoon and dip it in the butter. Pour that onto a portion of your plate. This way you will only be adding a teaspoon or so of butter to your shellfish.

6. When visiting your friendly neighborhood deli, avoid selecting the corned beef, pastrami, sausage, liverwurst, bologna, meatloaf, or lun-

cheon meat sandwich (or mayo-drenched shrimp, tuna, or egg salad sandwiches). Choose instead sandwiches filled with chicken or turkey breast, cheese, or roast beef, and try to wet the bread with mustard or a teeny bit of mayo (about half a teaspoon).

7. On the side, load up on complex carbohydrates, such as rice pilaf, veggies, beans, or boiled or baked potatoes.

8. What about the tempting dessert tray? Of course, being satisfied with a bowl of fresh fruit would be great, but is it realistic all the time? If the fruit comes complete with whipped cream, ask them to dab a little dollop on top (not plop a pile all over). For those times when you just can't hold yourself back from the Chocolate Whiskey Cake or Hot Apple Pie, order one slice and share it with someone. Keep in mind most pies and pastries are actually higher in fat than cakes (except cakes with extra thick layers of filling or frosting). Angel food cake is the lowest fat cake of all.

For Better or For Worse: Menu Selections

So many choices—Chinese or Japanese, basic Italian or just pizza, should we go Mexican and Margaritas or French and red wine? And once you choose "where" to go, you still have to decide "what" to order.

For example, most people don't picture 650 calories (77 percent from fat) alongside the vision of one slice of Quiche Lorraine dancing in their heads as they drive to their favorite French restaurant.

And if you're an avid lover of Fettucine Alfredo, sorry Charlie, but it's time to cut the courtship. Alfredo, dressed in the typical Italian fare, is carrying a bit of excess fat with him, to say the least. He has 720 calories per serving with 81 percent from fat. No cause for panic though. You can still make it a lower fat (and still delicious) way at home.

Let's take an up-close and personal look at some international favorites, as well as a couple more American options.

French

While thumbing through my *Mastering the Art of French Cooking* cookbook by Julia Child, I couldn't help but notice that if you have to describe the "art of French cooking" in four words or less, they would be "eggs, butter, cream, and salt." They are in almost every recipe. It seems the only way to get away from them is to move to another country.

We might all expect the standard light and fluffy cheese souffle to be loaded with fat and cholesterol (a two-cup serving has about 600 calories, 70 percent from fat and almost 500 milligrams of cholesterol). But what about a seemingly innocent menu item described as "scallops with wine, garlic, and herbs?" In this case, the menu failed to inform the eater it also contains butter, olive oil, and cheese. And don't let those elegant names sidetrack you, such as lobster thermidor, which happens to be laced with butter and whipping cream.

So enough of the bad news. The key to eating healthful but still eating French is "Watch Your Sauces." You can start off with a lean chicken breast or fish fillet, but given a chance the French will smother it in a heavy sauce like Hollandaise or Bernaise (made with egg yolks and butter), which has about 450 calories per half cup (98 percent from fat), 250 milligrams of cholesterol, and about 750 milligrams of sodium. Bechamel sauce (made with milk, butter, and flour) has 228 calories per half cup, with 74 percent from fat, and 57 milligrams of cholesterol, plus about 900 milligrams of sodium.

You can either ask that only one tablespoon of these sauces be added to your fish or chicken or you can order (or cook) your entree with a Bordelaise sauce (wine sauce), which has about 155 calories per half cup. About 76 percent of the calories are from fat, and Bordelaise sauce has only about 10 milligrams of cholesterol and 400 milligrams of sodium.

There are unadulterated French recipes that actually come to your table already pretty low in fat, such as steamed mussels or fish fillets poached in white wine. The latter has 227 calories per serving, with 26 percent of calories from fat, 125 milligrams of cholesterol, and about 220 milligrams of sodium.

What about crepes? Well, I confess, I'm a crepe lover from way back. Just remember, before you decide what to fill it or top it with, one crepe (all by itself) starts off with 150 calories, 40 percent from fat, and 100 milligrams of cholesterol.

Italian

If I could eat my way through any country, it would be Italy, no question. Mostly because of the two "P" words—Pizza and Pasta. (I don't care what the food critics say. In my book, pasta is still "IN.")

I know, pizza is different over there. Actually it's probably lower in fat because they like their pizza dough with only a little cheese on it (unlike us Americans who like our cheese with only a little pizza bread under it). But even if you have it the American way, if you order the vegetarian special or cheese only versions (no extra cheese), you're still dealing with a comparatively low-fat entree (28 to 32 percent of calories from fat).

In the pasta department, one of your best choices is mushroom spaghetti. Even the stand-by spaghetti and meatballs isn't too bad—with 38 percent of calories from fat. If you're going to cover your noodles or ravioli with something, choose the Marsala, made with wine, or Marinara, made with tomatoes, onions, and garlic. It's the pesto and cream type sauces that are the troublemakers. Mix your fettucini noodles with a pesto cream sauce and suddenly you're looking at a 67 percent calories from fat dish.

If it's a must-have situation, you could order or serve your pasta with half the original amount of sauce. This will cut the fat and calories way down.

Then comes a dilemma I know I've faced in a few Italian restaurants: Manicotti or cannelloni, which should it be?

Well, the answer is neither—at least not the way they're traditionally made. Both have about 800 calories a serving (namely, two manicotti or cannelloni rolls), with 65 percent of calories from fat and from 300 to 600 milligrams of cholesterol. But you could order or serve them covered with a Marinara sauce and just a sprinkle of cheese—instead of the creamy sauces and blankets of cheese usually topping them.

You will get less stuffing and more pasta for your money when you stuff a ravioli or tortellini instead of a cannelloni—one of the best ways I know to lower the percent of fat calories. A large serving of meat-filled ravioli with a tomato sauce and a generous amount of cheese has around 700 calories, with 42 percent from fat.

With a last name like Moquette, my European bias toward food may come as no surprise. Still, I do love foods from the South and East as well. First, we'll look at some Mexican Cuisine.

Mexican

The first choice confronting anyone planning a Tex-Mex type meal is flour versus corn tortillas. They are different in more ways than just color. The flour-type has the four-letter "L" word in it—LARD.

Flour tortillas have up to 150 calories each, compared with corn tortillas with about 50 calories. The flour types have 34 percent of calories from fat, compared with 10 percent for corn tortillas. Flour tortillas have about 140 milligrams of sodium, while corn tortillas have just one milligram of sodium each. Deep fry either one, though, and it doesn't matter which you've chosen. They'll both come up loaded with grease and calories. So it's best to leave those entrees with fried tortillas where they belong—on the menu!

The second major consideration, especially when dining out, is whether to reach into that basket of tortilla chips or to hold off until dinner. One innocent handful of chips adds about 140 calories, half of which are from fat. And dip them into the salsa or chili sauces? One-fourth cup contains around 900 milligrams of sodium!

If you have a thing for that chili-flavored sausage, chorizo, try and forget about it. A small 2-ounce serving has about 430 calories, 83 percent from fat, and 85 milligrams of cholesterol. And, speaking of fat and cholesterol, a typical recipe of Huevos Rancheros has 530 milligrams of cholesterol—480 calories, 50 percent from fat, and about 2,000 milligrams of sodium. You're already way past your daily cholesterol target of 300 milligrams a day and darn near your sodium limit of 3,000 milligrams. And you haven't even left the breakfast table!

So what can you order or cook up? Believe it or not, that side of rice and beans, even the refried type, is a good place to start. Even though the secret "refried" ingredient is usually lard (they have cans of "vegetarian refried beans" that add vegetable oil instead), a typical 3/4-cup side serving with a sprinkle of melted Jack cheese on top is still between 25 and 35 percent of calories from fat—around 300 calories, with 20 milligrams of cholesterol, 100 milligrams of sodium, and an impressive 15 grams of fiber!! Not bad!

The distinctively Mexican tomato-colored rice has about 240 calories per 3/4-cup serving, with 22 percent of calories from fat. Depending on the recipe, the rice can have up to 600 milligrams of sodium.

For possible entrees, I'll give it to you straight:

- Try to order them without the sour cream or guacamole. Per 1/4-cup dollop, sour cream has 125 calories, 86 percent from fat, and 32 milligrams of cholesterol. Guacamole has almost 100 calories per 1/4 cup, with 79 percent from fat (but no cholesterol).

- If you absolutely have to have the taco or tostada, order chicken instead of beef and ask if you can have it with a baked or steamed tortilla instead of fried. (Don't tell yourself "it's the best part," because it isn't. And even if you think it is, it's not worth all the extra fat and calories.)

- Chicken tends to be the lowest fat enchilada (about 35 percent of calories from fat and around 240 calories each, 30 milligrams of cholesterol, and 200 milligrams of sodium).

- If you're a burrito person:

—Bean burritos are always a safe bet (about 30 percent fat calories from a total of 340 calories, 7.5 grams of fiber, 7 milligrams of cholesterol, and 270 milligrams of sodium).

—The beef and bean combos (about 36 percent calories from fat) are usually better choices than the all-beef types.

—Those fresh, regular-sized vegetarian burritos (where they, or you, fill a steamed tortilla with whole beans, rice, mild salsa, and some cheese) are an excellent choice. I indulge in these at least once a week. One, which is usually more than plenty for me, has about 500 calories, 20 percent from fat, 11 grams of fiber, and 26 milligrams of cholesterol. Sodium values can get up around 1,300 milligrams, depending on the chili sauce and how much you or they add. The one with chicken but no cheese is still a great choice. It has about the same calories, percent of fat calories, and fiber as the vegetarian—but twice the cholesterol.

- What's the secret to these soft, yummy cornmeal tamale exteriors? They're held together with lots of LARD! (There's that word again!) So don't be shocked that half the calories are from fat. The chicken ones are pretty low in calories (around 300 for two small tamales), so technically you could probably have a low-fat meal if you ate some rice and enough fruit or something to bring down the percentage of calories from fat. The same goes for chicken tacos. Two have about 300 calories, 40 percent from fat.

- And here's my last word on eating Mexican. Think twice—or even three times—before opting for a cheesy chili relleno. One dinky relleno has 500 calories, 62 percent of calories from fat, 185 milligrams of cholesterol, and up to 1,500 milligrams of sodium.

Chinese

Let's start off by listing some of the more obvious no-no's. Fried wontons, fried noodles, fried egg rolls, Egg Foo Young (66 percent of calories from fat and 400 milligrams of cholesterol per serving), too much soy sauce or teriyaki sauce (a mere 1/4 teaspoon of soy sauce has 100 milligrams of sodium). And if you're in a restaurant, ask if your food can be made without monosodium glutamate.

Not so obvious no-no's:

It's best to avoid lobster sauce, which contains egg yolks, fried rice, which typically adds up to 400 calories a cup, with 45 percent of calories from fat, Peking duck, crispy fish (which is crispy because it's fried), batter dipped and fried shrimp or chicken, and fried dim sum appetizers.

Before we go any further, I have just three words to emphasize: *Eat your rice.* Rice is your salvation from ordering high or moderately high-fat stir-fry dishes. You see, rice has a glorious 237 calories per cup—almost all complex carbohydrate calories (91 percent) and only 2 percent fat calories. Can't beat those numbers!

So say you order green pepper beef or Mongolian beef (where the mixture is mostly beef strips). How much rice are we talking about? A good rule to follow if your entree is mostly meat is to add about twice as much rice as your meat dish. I'll show you how it works. Say you're looking down at 3/4 cup green pepper beef (at 285 calories, 68 percent from fat). If you add or mix it with 1 1/2 cups rice, the meal is now 28 percent calories from fat.

If you're dealing with a mixture that is about half chicken, tofu, or meat and the other half vegetables, you'll only need to add the same amount of rice as your stir-fry dish. Take broccoli with chicken (a 1 1/4-cup serving has 267 calories, 47 percent from fat), plop it over 1 1/4 cup rice, and suddenly it's a 23-percent-calories-from-fat meal, with 563 total calories. You would follow this rule whether you chose shrimp in black bean sauce, tofu with veggies, chicken in snow peas, or whatever, as long as part of the dish was definitely vegetables.

Well, thanks for listening. You may have undergone a shock or two. But if it makes you feel any better, I underwent one of my own. I had no idea Mu Shu Pork (you know, that wonderful dish with mushrooms, scrambled egg, etc., all wrapped up in a cute little Chinese crepe-like pancake with hoisin sauce and green onion strips) was so high in percent of calories from fat (about 46 percent)! It's reasonably low in calories (2 pancakes stuffed have about 275 calories), so it's possible to make it "part" of a low-fat meal. Still, that 46 percent was a shock!

Japanese

Once again, when you choose Japanese, stay away from the deep-fried dishes such as tempura, tonkatsu (deep fried pork), torikatsu (deep fried chicken), and katsudon (deep fried pork, onion, and egg). And keep the high-sodium sauces to a minimum. In fact, ask for them on the side. Just 3 teaspoons of teriyaki sauce adds 700 milligrams of sodium—but zero fat and only 15 calories.

The key words on a Japanese menu are "yakimono" which means broiled with little fat added and "rice," your low-fat, go-with-anything, carbohydrate-rich filler.

Speaking of rice, are we voting "yes" on sushi? (This new taste sensation, although not new to the Japanese, is vinegared rice rolled up several different ways, including with seaweed, and combined with raw fish or vegetables or both.) Yes. Yes. And triple yes. There is no added fat involved in sushi making. Even when an oily raw fish is used, it's more as a decoration, such as a strip of fish acting as a center in a seaweed roll or a thin fillet laying atop a bed of rice.

Tofu is a great meat alternative, if you're into those, with 4 ounces (about 1/2 cup) totalling 81 calories, 40 percent from protein, and no cholesterol. It is 48 percent calories from fat, but at 81 calories, you won't do much damage to your percentage from fat for the meal. If we were talking about the same amount of relatively lean beef (2 1/2 ounces), for example, we would be dealing instead with about 53 percent of calories from fat and 185 added calories.

Greek

What can I say. The Greeks like their meat, olive oil, butter, and creamy dressings. What I remember clearest of this Greek restaurant I went to in Holland (which I figured was "more authentic" than the ones I had gone to here, since the Dutch and the Greeks at least share the same continent) was that I have never seen as much cooked meat on one plate before in my entire life. They literally "piled" it on. So the first suggestion I have is to keep your meat portion modest. There is an ancient proverb (that I just made up) that says: "The meat you take home tonight could fill tomorrow's sandwich."

I also recall a smaller, creamier pile lying conveniently next to the meat pile and resembling mayonnaise. Remember, 1/4 cup is equal to 400 calories, 98 percent from fat! A yogurt dressing (there is a type mixed with garlic and cucumbers called Tzatziki) would cost you fewer calories, but since it's probably made from whole milk, it would still be at least 47 percent calories from fat. If you're making it at home, use the nonfat or low-fat plain yogurts.

Also, keep the anchovies, olives, and feta cheese in perspective. All three are high in percent of calories from fat and in sodium. (Six olives contain 50 calories, 93 percent from fat, plus 230 milligrams of sodium. Three anchovies equal 25 calories, 54 percent of them from fat. Two ounces of feta cheese have 150 calories, 71 percent from fat, and 632 milligrams of sodium.)

One Greek taste treat rates in the "very high-fat" category—probably the richest dessert cake ever created, *baklava*. Before you take the first bite, just promise me you'll think about the pound of butter (4 sticks!), 2 pounds of naturally fat nuts, 2 cups of honey, and 2 cups of sugar that went into the baklava.

Hang in there. I'm almost finished with the "bad" list. Avoid ordering babaganoosh (an eggplant appetizer made with fat), Kibbeh (lamb and butter), and those two wonderfully fatty pies, Tyropita and Spanokopita.

So, what's left? The forever famous shish kabob, where lamb and assorted vegetables are broiled on a spit, or Plaki, fish cooked with tomatoes, onions, and garlic. And you can have plenty of pilaf, rice, and bread— as long as you go extremely easy on the butter.

Deli Delights

Sandwiches—the one common noon-hour notion that often makes its way onto our dinner plates and into our picnic baskets. Not to worry though, sandwiches can be a healthful alternative to greasy fast food, frozen entrees, or the usual picnic munchies such as fried chicken or barbecued hot dogs. You just have to know what to fill them with and how to dress them up.

There's a huge difference healthwise between a French-dip steak sandwich with mayo dripping down the sides and a breast of turkey sandwich on wheat with spicy mustard and juicy tomato slices. And it's much better to eat a chicken breast sandwich with no mayonnaise or butter (about 16 percent calories from fat) than a chicken salad sandwich (about 48 percent of calories from fat). See what I mean? So on to the sandwich suggestions.

Suggestion #1.

Start with a low-fat bread—preferably something high in fiber. Choose the whole wheat or whole grain types or even sourdough, but leave the croissants, crescent rolls, or other fancy fatty breads for someone else.

Suggestion #2.

Choose a lower-fat filling. The more desirable fillers are turkey or chicken breast slices (about 19 percent calories from fat), roast beef slices (24 percent calories from fat), or tuna, chicken, shrimp, and crab salad, made with yogurt or small amounts of reduced-calorie mayonnaise. The world's worst fillers are salami (75 percent calories from fat), Polish sausage or liverwurst (80 percent fat calories), bologna (82 percent fat calories), and chicken, tuna, and egg salad with regular mayonnaise (71, 76, and 87 percent calories from fat, respectively).

Suggestion #3.

Add all the lettuce leaves, tomato slices, and onion rings you want. They'll add no more than 10 calories each. I must confess, avocado and turkey is one of my favorite sandwiches, so it is with great pain that I announce to you that one-third of an avocado adds about 110 calories (79 percent from fat).

Suggestion #4.

Lay off the mayonnaise. In case you hadn't heard, just one tablespoon of mayonnaise (which is about the amount that globs onto your knife after you pull it from the jar) adds 100 calories, 98 percent of which are from fat. This, of course, can make or break your sandwich's goal of "no more than 30 percent of calories from fat."

Try adding some color instead—yellow or red. One teaspoon of mustard adds less than 5 calories and 65 milligrams of sodium, while one tablespoon of catsup adds about 18 calories and 170 milligrams of sodium.

Suggestion #5.

Pass up the mayonnaise-coated potato salads and coleslaws. One cup of standard potato salad has almost 400 calories (67 percent from fat) and 190 milligrams of cholesterol. One cup of cole slaw has 150 calories, with 63 percent from fat. Keep your sandwich company with a fruit or vegetable salad, or a green salad with reduced fat dressing.

Suggestion #6.

Skip the chips. When you grab each little bag of chips (about 2 ounces), you're buying about 325 extra calories (with 62 percent from fat) and 350 milligrams of sodium.

I hope these suggestions haven't taken the fun out of fixing or ordering yourself a sandwich.

Salad Bar Savvy

We opt for the salad bar, thinking to ourselves, "I'll be good today." Or we drag others to the best salad bar in town instead of Hamburger Heaven, promptly explaining that we're "on a diet" or that we're "watching it."

What we don't realize is that when we confidently line up at that salad bar, we're really skipping through a virtual fat and calorie minefield.

I'm going to describe a typical salad bar meal, and you tell me whether it comes close to your salad bar expectations.

You start out with about 2 cups of crisp and crunchy lettuce. (You try to pick out the real green leaves, but there are usually only a few left.) Then you grab a few cherry tomatoes and some sliced cucumber, a spoon of chopped egg and bacon, several strips of ham, maybe a scoop (about 1/4 cup) of grated cheddar cheese, and two small ladles or about 1/4 cup total of dressing. (A lot of people use twice this amount.)

Then, just when you thought there was no possible way you could fit one more thing into your salad bowl, you spot the chunky potato salad and the creamy macaroni salad. So you manage to balance about 1/3 cup of each on the side of the bowl. You've just walked away from the salad bar carrying a total of 775 calories—75 percent from FAT. Sound like a diet plate to you?

The point is you CAN eat a wonderfully low-fat, high-fiber, tasty meal at a salad bar. You just have to have some savvy. You have to know what to sprinkle on top of your salad and what to skip. You need to learn which spoons to keep your hands off of and which to use freely. As a guide, take a look for yourself at the accompanying chart.

Choose the Most Healthful Salad Ingredients

Salad Ingredients 1/8 cup portions unless otherwise noted	% Calories from fat	Calories	Fiber (grams)
Maximize these:			
cauliflower, 1/3 cup	less than 10%	4	0.5
carrot, grated	less than 10%	5	0.5
strawberries/pineapple, 1/3 cup	less than 10%	15-50	1.0
melon pieces, 1/3 cup	less than 10%	20	0.5
kidney beans	less than 10%	27	2.0
green peas	less than 10%	12	2.0
tomato, 1/2 whole	less than 10%	12	1.0
cucumber, 6 slices	less than 10%	2	—
broccoli, 1/3 cup	less than 10%	8	2.0
green pepper	less than 10%	4	—
crab meat and shrimp, 1/3 cup	less than 20%	40-60	—
mushrooms	less than 20%	2	0.5
garbanzo beans	less than 20%	30	1.3
turkey/chicken breast, 1/3 cup	less than 20%	70-80	—

Salad Ingredients	% Calories from fat	Calories	Fiber (grams)
1/8 cup portions unless otherwise noted			

Minimize these:

Salad Ingredients	% Calories from fat	Calories	Fiber (grams)
lean ham, 1/3 cup diced	37%	68	—
fried noodles, croutons	43%	28	—
coleslaw, 1/3 cup	55%	120	0.5
Parmesan cheese	60%	44	—
chopped egg	65%	16	—
potato salad, 1/3 cup	67%	128	1.0
sunflower seeds	71%	97	1.0
macaroni salad, 1/3 cup	74%	118	—
cheddar cheese, grated	74%	55	—
bacon, crumbled, 1 Tbsp	78%	18	—
avocado, 1/4 whole	79%	81	1.5
black olives	93%	25	1.0

Dress for Success Tips:

- Too much of any dressing defeats the purpose of a healthy salad. Try to dress your salad with only 2 to 3 tablespoons.

- Fruit juices, vinegars, and herbs make dressings flavorful without adding fat or salt.

- For guilt-free creamy dressings, use buttermilk or lower fat yogurt and add reduced calorie mayonnaise sparingly to thicken it.

- For a tangy fruit salad topping, try low-fat yogurt such as vanilla or lemon.

Dressings:	% Calories from fat	Calories
(2 Tablespoons)		

Maximize these:

Dressings:	% Calories from fat	Calories
nonfat yogurt, plain	3%	16
low-fat yogurt, flavored	9%	29
low-fat yogurt, plain	22%	18
light sour cream	60%	45

Dressings: (2 Tablespoons)	% Calories from fat	Calories
Minimize these:		
Reduced calorie		
mayo-type dressings	73%	70
Thousand island	83%	118
French	84%	134
Russian	90%	151
Italian	91%	137
Bleu cheese	91%	154
Ranch	92%	109

The first thing you can do is pick the right greens. Spinach has more than four times the fiber and vitamin A and three times the vitamin C of all the other types of lettuce. Your best choice after that is Romaine and leaf lettuce, which have more vitamin A, C, and calcium than the others.

Then, when you've got the nutrient-rich bed of lettuce ready, you don't want to ruin it by adding all sorts of fat, cholesterol, and sodium. That means skipping the crocks of chopped egg, bacon, croutons, fried noodles, grated cheese, sliced olives, avocado, and creamy salads, such as potato salad and macaroni salads.

Instead, dip all you want into the green peas, beets, sliced mushrooms, kidney and garbanzo beans, tomato, sliced cucumber, green pepper strips, grated carrot, broccoli, and cauliflower. You can usually get away with a tablespoon or so of grated Parmesan or cheddar cheese and you can add some shrimp, crab meat, or turkey. Lay low on the sliced ham. It's usually higher in fat and sodium than the others.

Just by adding 1/8 cup each of peas, kidney beans, and broccoli, the fiber in your salad is up to 6 grams. You're also well on your way to meeting the recommended daily requirement for certain vitamins and minerals. For example, just by adding 1/3 cup broccoli, you're already halfway to your vitamin C requirement.

Now that you've carefully constructed a perfectly healthful salad, you must choose a dressing and how much of that dressing just as judiciously. Somewhere between French and Thousand Island, Italian dressing deceitfully became the lower fat dressing of choice. As you can see from the evidence in the accompanying table, they're all pretty much the same. Italian dressing has just as much fat and just as many calories as the others.

The only way to be able to add more than a few drops of dressing to your mound of foliage is to use the reduced-calorie types. Wishbone Reduced Calorie Lite Ranch has 40 calories per tablespoon and 3 grams of fat, compared with the regular Ranch, which has 80 calories and twice the fat. Bernstein's Reduced Calorie Italian with Cheese dressing has only 8 calories per tablespoon and less than one gram of fat.

But don't get too crazy with the reduced-calorie types. The ones with 40 calories per tablespoon can add up quickly and the others with about 10 calories per tablespoon come with quite a bit of sodium.

On a salad with 2 cups of spinach or Romaine leaves, a few cherry tomatoes, 1/3 cup broccoli, and crab, 1/8 cup of sliced mushrooms, garbanzo beans, and green pepper, for example, if you drizzle 1 tablespoon of reduced calorie ranch dressing, you'll end up with a 195 calorie salad, with 36 percent of calories from fat. If you use Bernstein's Italian Dressing, it's a 125 calorie salad with 13 percent of calories from fat.

If the salad bar is your entire meal, obviously less than 200 calories isn't going to cut it. So load up on items like beans, peas, shrimp, or turkey, broccoli and cauliflower, etc. And, don't forget the fresh fruit that some salad bars offer for dessert.

The All American Diner and Coffee Shop

Wherever you are in the United States, there's one type of restaurant you'll find just about everywhere—the American-style diner and coffee shop. It could be Lou's Diner or the Pennsylvania Pancake House. But no matter what it's called, you'll usually find fixings such as pancakes, waffles, potatoes, and eggs served during the morning hours and burgers, grilled cheese sandwiches, and steaks served until closing.

Even at the diner in your town, or the town you're passing through, there are lower fat choices awaiting you.

Better Breakfast Selections

- Two pieces of toast or one English muffin with 1 teaspoon of butter = 200 calories, 25 percent from fat, 11 milligrams of cholesterol, and 400 milligrams of sodium.

- Two pieces of toast or one English muffin with 1 teaspoon butter and 1 tablespoon of jam and preserves = 250 calories, 25 percent from fat, 11 milligrams of cholesterol, and 400 milligrams of sodium.

- One medium-sized biscuit made from a mix, with 2 teaspoons of jam or preserves = 180 calories, 27 percent from fat, 54 milligrams of cholesterol, and 375 milligrams of sodium.

- Hot or cold cereal (see cereal section for listing of low-fat choices in "Supermarket Savvy" chapter). Ask for skim or low-fat milk. These are sometimes served with fresh fruit, too!

- Full stack (3) of pancakes with 2 tablespoons of syrup = 280 calories, 18 percent from fat, with 60 milligrams of cholesterol, and 265 milligrams of sodium.

- French toast (2 pieces and 2 tablespoons of syrup) = 370 calories, 22 percent from fat (33 percent without syrup), 145 milligrams of cholesterol, and 400 milligrams of sodium.

- Three pancakes with 2 tablespoons syrup and 2 slices of bacon = 355 calories, 28 percent from fat, 70 milligrams of cholesterol, and 570 milligrams of sodium.

The "You Could Order Worse" Breakfast Selections

- Strawberry waffle with 1/4 cup whipped cream = 495 calories, 33 percent from fat, 95 milligrams cholesterol, and 370 milligrams of sodium.

- Pigs in a blanket (3 pancakes, 3 sausage links, and 2 tablespoons syrup, but no butter) = 425 calories, 37 percent from fat, 90 milligrams cholesterol, and 870 milligrams of sodium.

- Three strawberry pancakes with 1/4 cup whipped cream = 465 calories, 31 percent from fat, 95 milligrams cholesterol, and 360 milligrams of sodium.
- One medium blueberry muffin = 225 calories, 30 percent from fat, 40 milligrams cholesterol, and 350 milligrams sodium.
- One medium bran muffin = 210 calories, 30 percent from fat, 42 milligrams cholesterol, and 355 milligrams sodium.

Better Lunch/Dinner Selections

(For sandwich selections, refer to the Deli Delights section.)

- One medium baked potato with 1 teaspoon butter = 180 calories, 20 percent from fat, 10 milligrams cholesterol, and 45 milligrams sodium.

OR

One medium baked potato with 2 tablespoons sour cream = 205 calories, 25 percent from fat, 15 milligrams cholesterol, and 20 milligrams sodium.

OR

One medium baked potato with 1 teaspoon butter and 1 tablespoon sour cream = 210 calories, 29 percent from fat, 20 milligrams cholesterol, and 50 milligrams sodium.

- One cup of chili with beans (no cheese) and a slice of French bread (no butter) = 400 calories, 34 percent from fat, 38 milligrams cholesterol, and up to 1,300 milligrams of sodium, depending on whether or not it's canned.
- A quarter-pound hamburger on a large bun with no mayonnaise or cheese added (catsup or mustard optional) = 400 calories, about 40 percent from fat, 75 milligrams cholesterol, and 470 milligrams sodium.
- Choice sirloin steak (9 1/2 ounces raw) with 2 slices of French bread (1 teaspoon butter) and 1 cup of vegetables = 660 calories, 30 percent from fat, 195 milligrams cholesterol, and 530 milligrams sodium—if no salt is added to the steak.

Some Items That Might Surprise You

- Huevos Rancheros (flour tortilla with ground beef and beans, scrambled eggs, cheese, and salsa) = 650 calories, 60 percent from fat, 600 milligrams cholesterol, and more than 1,000 milligrams of sodium.

- One hot dog or corn dog with mustard = 325 calories, 56 percent from fat, 35 milligrams of cholesterol, and 1,050 to 1,250 milligrams of sodium.

- One slice apple pie (1/6 of a 9-inch pie) = 400 calories, 38 percent from fat, 475 milligrams of sodium.

- Bacon versus sausage "on the side:"

  One strip of bacon has 35 calories, 56 percent from fat, 5 milligrams of cholesterol, and 100 milligrams of sodium.

  One link sausage has 48 calories, 77 percent from fat, 10 milligrams of cholesterol, and 170 milligrams of sodium.

- Grilled cheese sandwich = 400 calories, 55 percent from fat, 55 milligrams of cholesterol, and 1,150 milligrams of sodium.

The lesson here is that it IS indeed possible to eat out in restaurants and maintain a low-fat diet. Of course, each restaurant will be preparing their items in their own special way. Some chefs might have a heavier hand when it comes to pouring oil or cream, for example. But for the purposes of this chapter, customary recipes were used for the computer analysis and should encompass most establishments today.

Before we leave this subject though, I want to remind you that the survival of any restaurant depends on whether or not they have customers to serve. And whether or not customers return to a restaurant depends on how pleased they were with their meal and dining experience. You hold all the cards. If you want your fish broiled without added butter, if you want your sandwich prepared without mayonnaise, then it's in the restaurant's best business interest to serve it to you that way. So don't be afraid to ask how something is prepared or to request that it be prepared a little differently just for you.

Dine Smart—Dine Lean

Okay, so I know you read the whole chapter, just to have me add a simple summary at the end that will really "sum" it all up. If you want to be sure to eat healthy when you are eating out, here are my two keys for success:

1. Select the right restaurant. Make sure you go to a restaurant that offers some low-fat entrees or is at least willing to prepare yours without the fat.
2. Select the right menu item(s).

That should be easy enough, right? Now here are some questions to ask your waiter. Remember that it never hurts to ask. The only thing you stand to lose is some extra fat and calories.

1. How is this prepared?
2. Is there any butter or oil added?
3. Is this made with mayonnaise?
4. Is this made with cream?
5. Can this be steamed, grilled, or broiled instead of fried?
6. Can I have the sauce/dressing on the side?
7. Can this be cooked in wine or broth instead of butter or oil?
8. Can you remove the skin from my chicken before it's prepared?
9. Can I substitute a salad, baked potato, or steamed vegetables for the french fries?

So, there you have it. Everything you need to know before you dine-around.

Chapter 6

Grab A Bite And Run

The great part about "eating in" is that YOU get to be the chef! "Great," you say, "I never asked to be a chef." But think about it: It's the chef and only the chef who controls "what" and "how much" is added to make the meal. When you eat in, YOU choose whether yogurt or sour cream is added to your chicken enchilada, whether your fish fillet is simmered in wine or butter, whether you shake basil and pepper onto your pasta instead of salt. YOU choose whether to follow a diet that meets disease prevention guidelines.

The Fight Fat Basics—A Survival Course

We've talked about how to cut the fat in foods that others prepare (fast food, food companies, restaurants, etc.). But what about food that we have no one to blame but ourselves, where WE actually perform the act of cutting the butter or pouring the oil? There are basically six steps to successfully cut the fat at home:

#1. *Beware of Mixers.* I'm referring to products we use to mix or dip other foods, such as mayonnaise, salad dressings, and sour cream.

#2. *Pay Attention to Naturally Fat Foods.* These foods are mostly fat themselves, such as cheese or some red meat. This doesn't mean they're "bad" foods. We just have to start treating them with some respect. You might begin by using smaller quantities, such as "sprinkling" cheese instead of "slicing" it in chunks.

#3. *Try Not to Eat Two Naturally Fat Foods Together.* This means not adding cheese to a high-fat cracker or ham sandwich or butter to a croissant, tartar sauce or mayonnaise to a fried fish fillet, etc.

#4. *Use Less Fat in the Preparation of Food.* Bake, oven broil (draining off any fat), boil, stew (skimming the fat off), poach, stir fry (without a lot of oil), simmer, or steam. Use nonstick cookware to avoid adding cooking fat. Substitute low-fat liquids, such as broth, tomato juice, lemon juice or wine, for grease in cooking.

#5. *Add Less Fat at the Table.* Be aware of these "table fats" and how much they're costing you. For example, next time you're staring down at that bare potato, remember sour cream is about 85 percent calories from fat and 26 calories per tablespoon, while nonfat plain yogurt is only about 3 percent calories from fat and 8 calories per tablespoon.

#6. *Add Fruits, Vegetables, and Grains.* Pasta and breads somehow have developed the reputation for being "fattening." But if you look at the facts—or fats—it isn't the complex carbohydrates at all but what we ADD to them that can quickly boost the calories from fat. One full cup of boiled noodles only has about 170 calories and is 10 percent calories from fat. Olive oil is 100 percent calories from fat, and two tablespoons will add 238 calories. A typical thick white sauce is 71 percent calories from fat, and 1/2 cup will add 262 calories.

You can even add a layer of pasta or vegetables to your main dish instead of other more fat-filled items. For example, use a layer of pasta instead of one of the layers of cheese for your lasagna, or cut the amount of meat used to make a spaghetti sauce or casserole in half by adding vegetables instead.

Equipment you might not have:

#1. Can you say "Teflon?" Save yourself from all the grease and shortening you usually need to coat your frying pan or baking tins to keep your food from sticking. Try non-stick Teflon. I know I sound like a commercial again, but honest, I don't own any stock in Teflon companies!

What I do own are quality, nonstick frying pans (one large and one small), bundt pans, a cookie sheet, loaf pans, muffin pans, and casserole dishes. Nonstick pans are wonderful for all kinds of foods, from pizza crust (without olive oil) to cakes (without shortening). But buy the best quality, bonded versus the spray-on types, so the surface doesn't wear off easily. Some are easy to scratch, too, so it's wise to use only plastic utensils. (And only use a plastic scrubber.)

#2. This next piece of equipment is going to cost a bit more—La Food Processor. Trust me, you'll be more likely to make meals and snacks from scratch with "Oscar" (or any other food processor) on your team.

For example, when whipping the Almost Fat-Free Dip/Dressing in Chapter 9, a food processor will work best. And to make the incredibly colorful and tasty Creamy Carrot Sauce in Chapter 8, not only will it make grating carrots easier, but it's essential for the puree part. Not to mention the delicious pasta or crepe filling recipe also found in Chapter 8, "Chicken, Basil, and Baby Carrot Filling," which definitely requires the pureeing advantages of a food processor.

#3. The novelty of the '80s, the Microwave Oven, is the necessity of the '90s.

How else can you cook potatoes in eight minutes flat? Low-fat leftovers are more likely to be eaten, at work or at home, when a microwave is present. Vegetables can be cooked a few minutes before your main dish is ready. Items can be defrosted at the last minute using a microwave. I even use the microwave to make the Two-Minute Cheese Sauce in Chapter 7.

How to Cut Corners in the Kitchen and Cut Fat Too!

Most of our family lives could be described as "busy" to say the least— what with parent-teacher nights, school fundraising events, taking the kids to karate or piano lessons. Not to mention working in the occasional aerobics class or golf game, reading to your toddler, or helping your school-age child with homework.

Usually the time required for these tasks is non-negotiable, but the time you spend cooking in the kitchen sure is. The desire and need to cut corners in the kitchen is at an all-time high. But being health-conscious, we know the premium for cutting fat in food is also at an all-time high.

Add to this the trend in palate preferences for homemade taste and old-fashioned foods and you have today's quandary: how to balance convenience with health and homemade flavors.

Luckily in 1994, more than ever before, when it comes to cutting corners in the kitchen, we're not necessarily talking about TV dinners or microwave meals. We can buy low-fat products that help us prepare our freshly made meal in minutes (products like bottled spaghetti sauce, grated reduced fat cheese, canned beans, etc.). And we can buy any number of mixes that make it easier to whip up many of our favorite foods without having to start completely from scratch (like cake mixes, pancake mixes, potato, rice, stuffing, and pasta mixes).

In most cases the mix directions tell us to add much more fat than is necessary. For example, you usually don't have to add any of the fat called for on a cake mix box (there usually are already 4 grams of fat per serving in the mix powder alone). Just make sure to replace the amount of oil you don't add with some oil-free moisture-providing ingredient, such as nonfat sour cream, applesauce, vanilla yogurt, or the like.

In the potato, rice, stuffing, and pasta mix category, you can definitely get away with adding half as much butter or margarine. Many of these products now offer lower fat or cholesterol-free instructions right on the box. In some cases, you can cut the fat way back and add only one tablespoon per mix. You may want to add a little light or nonfat sour cream or use a tad more milk to add some richness and creaminess, though.

What can you save with every tablespoon of butter that stays on the stick or every tablespoon of oil that stays in the bottle? One tablespoon of butter contributes 102 calories and 11.5 grams of fat to the food total and one tablespoon of oil contributes 119 calories and 13.5 grams of fat.

The following products can help shave time and fat from your family's meals:

Mixes

You can cut the fat in these mixes by adding less than the amount called for in the directions.

Noodle Roni

Stove Top Stuffing

Uncle Ben's Rice Mixes

Scalloped Potato Mixes

Powdered Mashed Potatoes

Kraft Macaroni and Cheese Mix

Cake Mixes

Muffin and Nut Bread Mixes

Incomplete Pancake and Waffle Mixes

Reduced-Fat Bisquick Mix

Convenient Products for Favorite Recipes

- Ragu Fino Italian Garlic and Basil Spaghetti Sauce (and other bottled spaghetti sauces with no more than 3 grams of fat per 4-ounce serving. See Chapter 3 for lists.)

- Ore Ida Home Style and Golden Crinkles Frozen Fries

- Ore Ida Frozen Mashed Potatoes (just add skim or low-fat milk)

- Egg Beaters Fat-Free Egg Substitute or similar

- Armanino Pesto (frozen in plastic tub)

- Pepperidge Farms bottled gravies (98% fat free)

- Fresh packaged Lite Ravioli and Tortellini (eg. Contadina)

- Fresh packaged Lite Italian Sauces (eg. Contadina)

- Lite salad dressing packets (eg. Hidden Valley Ranch Lite)

- Low-fat soups (see Chapter 3)

- Campbell's Healthy Request Cream of Mushroom, Chicken, Celery, and Broccoli condensed soups for use in casseroles

- Canned beans
- Grated reduced-fat and fat-free cheeses (such as Healthy Choice nonfat Mozzarella, grated)
- Homestyle flour tortillas (can be used as a quick crust for quiche)
- Pillsbury All Ready Pizza Crust
- Pillsbury Soft Breadsticks

Stocking Your Kitchen for a Lighter New Year

It's simple. If you stock your kitchen with low-fat foods and products, you are more likely to cook and create low-fat meals and snacks. In addition to the products listed above, there are several other products I must mention as fat-fighting staples because many can be used to replace some or all of the fat in recipes and others are lower fat versions of common ingredients in recipes.

Other Fight Fat & Win Staples:

- light and nonfat sour cream
- reduced fat mayonnaise
- light and nonfat cream cheese (eg., Philadelphia Free)
- Frigo Fat Free Truly Lite Nonfat Ricotta Cheese
- low sodium chicken and beef broth
- liqueurs for dessert and quick bread recipes
- nonalcoholic beer, wine, etc.
- flavored vinegars
- applesauce
- Molly McButter sprinkles
- low-fat and nonfat cottage cheese (whipped in food processor)

- nonfat plain yogurt and flavored low-fat yogurts (eg., lemon, vanilla)
- reduced fat cheeses (eg., Cracker Barrel Light Sharp Cheddar)
- Louis Rich Turkey Bacon
- Dairy Maid Light Spread (best tasting diet margarine)
- Parmesan cheese

Ten Kitchen Staples for Fighting Fat

While filling my shopping cart last week, I couldn't help but notice I definitely favor a particular group of food items. Not so coincidentally, they all happen to be staples for waging war against fat in the diet.

I call this select group "staples" because I make sure these items can be found at any one time in my kitchen—and for good reason. I use some of them regularly to replace fat in recipes (i.e., Herb-Ox Low Sodium Chicken Broth) and others are lower fat alternatives to usually fat foods that I happen to love, along with most of America (i.e., Kraft Light Monterey Jack Cheese, Bernstein's Reduced Calorie Italian Dressing).

You may recognize a couple of these if you've glanced at the recipes in the next several chapters because I tend to use them over and over again when creating new low-fat recipes. So without further ado, allow me to introduce you to the Ten Fighting-Fat Staples:

#1. Low-fat bottled spaghetti sauce. There are now several brands that carry sauces with 0 or 1 gram of fat per 1/2 cup. And there are even more with 2 or 3 grams of fat per 1/2 cup. I always have a jar in my refrigerator to spread on pizza crust, pour over pasta or eggplant Parmesan, baked potatoes, etc., or to mix with chili powder or salsa to make a quick Mexican-style sauce for enchiladas or quesadillas.

Are you ready to be impressed? Most bottled spaghetti sauces have up to 9 grams of fat per 1/2 cup. I found this out while I was desperately trying to find my favorite Ragu sauce in a Lake Tahoe supermarket—to no avail. So I started looking at the nutrition information labels of the other bottled spaghetti sauces and none of them came close to being as low in fat as my Ragu.

In case you were wondering if this story had a happy ending, I did finally find a jar of low-fat spaghetti sauce, so my ski trip was indeed off to a proper start with a high complex carbohydrate, low-fat spaghetti dinner.

#2. *Bernstein's Low-Calorie Italian Dressing* (or other reduced-calorie Italian dressings, equally as tasty but low in fat). I don't know who "Bernstein" is, but he or she sure makes a taste-filled low-calorie salad dressing. You can drizzle two tablespoons gloriously guilt-free over your pasta, vegetables, tuna, chicken, or shrimp salad, over your grilled chicken breast or fish, or even on your traditional green salad. A two-tablespoon serving only costs you 12 calories and less than one gram of fat, a small price to pay for a versatile, delicious dressing. (Be careful, though, the sodium is still high at 275 milligrams per tablespoon.)

#3. *Herb-Ox Low Sodium Chicken Broth* (or other low-sodium chicken broths). How can chicken broth be a staple? Well, chicken broth is to me what vegetable oil or olive oil is to other people. I use it to stir fry, sauté vegetables, pan simmer fish or chicken fillets, boil and flavor rice, etc.

The broth comes in individual serving packets. You can make one cup at a time, which is great for people living alone or in pairs. One packet, or one cup of made-up broth, only adds 5 milligrams of sodium, while your run-of-the-mill broth or bouillon cube adds 800 milligrams.

#4. *Part-skim ricotta cheese.* This is a new staple for me. I've recently been discovering all sorts of wonderful ways to use it. I add it to Marinara sauce to make the sauce thicker and creamier. I use it as a base for my low-fat garlic spread on bread and for my low-fat cheese sauce. The cheese sauce can be used in casseroles, to perk up pasta, to top a potato, etc.

#5. *Aunt Jemima's Buttermilk, Whole Wheat, or Buckwheat Pancake and Waffle Mix* (the "incomplete" mixes). I couldn't talk about staples without talking about dear old Aunt Jemima. I mix her incomplete (which means you add the eggs, milk, and oil) buttermilk mix with her buckwheat mix to make semi-wheaty, fluffy pancakes or waffles. Don't follow the directions on the box, though. Just add egg whites and skim or low-fat milk. You don't need to add any oil or egg yolks.

#6. *Part-skim cheeses.* If I'm not adding an ounce of part-skim cheese to my toasted bagel in the morning, I'm grating some into my enchilada or pasta at dinner time. By grating Kraft Light Monterey Jack instead of regular cheeses, for example, I cut the fat by two-thirds! Most cheeses have about 9 grams of fat per ounce; others calling themselves "reduced fat" cheeses may have 7 or 8 grams of fat per ounce (check those labels). Those "part skim" mozzarella balls have around 5 grams of fat per ounce, and they definitely help bring down the fat. But Kraft's Light Monterey Jack, as well as their cheddar, has 3 grams of fat per ounce.

#7. *Skim milk.* Aside from its more typical reputation as a beverage, skim milk is a savvy substitute for many of the fatty ingredients usually called for in recipes, namely cream and whole milk. I add skim milk to make my "Very Berry Smoothie" or Salad Bar Quiche. It even teams up with part-skim ricotta cheese to make a low-fat cheese sauce or with plain nonfat yogurt to make an almost fat-free ranch dressing and dip.

#8. *Wine.* Ever wonder what you are possibly going to do with the bottles of wine that were "such a good deal, you had to buy them," yet tend not to use? Well, start wiping the dust off, because wine is a nice substitute for cooking fats and oils. I use wine to simmer mushrooms and onions instead of butter, margarine, or oils. I would say sauté instead of simmer, but this particular word specifically denotes the use of fat. However, where it says "sauté in butter or oil" in recipes, you can go ahead and use a nonfat ingredient such as wine.

#9. *Naturally butter flavored sprinkles.* For a butter lover such as myself, items like Molly McButter, Best O'Butter, or Butter Buds, where they extract the natural butter flavor and mix it with starch to create sprinkles, come in handy. I admit I have a hard time eating corn without a little butter, but the butter flavored sprinkles help me keep the calories in a reasonable range. For example, I use it to add some rich flavor to my favorite garlic spread recipe. You still need to watch the amount you add because 1/2 teaspoon may only add about 60 milligrams of sodium, but a tablespoon will add almost 400!

#10. Crackermeal. Cracker who? You may not have heard of or noticed this product on your supermarket shelf, but it's a staple in my kitchen because it's the "no fat added, no salt added" substitute for bread crumbs. Crackermeal can be used for coating your oven roasted chicken breast or fish fillet, as filler for your low-fat meat loaf or meatballs, and as topping for your low-fat fruit crisps and casseroles.

You didn't know breadcrumbs even had fat? If you read the label, you'll find most bread crumbs have a fat listed as the second ingredient and salt as the third!

A Few Words on Two Favorite Fatty Ingredients (Cheese and Beef)

The Big Cheese

All those in favor of cheese say "aye." All opposed? It's no secret, Americans definitely love their cheese, and lots of it. Sheets of cheese cover America's hamburgers, sandwiches, and hot dogs. Gobs of cheese sauce drip over piles of nacho chips and vegetables.

Me? Well, it's hard for me personally to imagine life without cheese. It's an irreplaceable ingredient on two of my favorite foods—lasagna and pizza. Where would eggplant be without Parmesan? Burger without cheese? Quiche without Lorraine? What would happen if enchiladas suddenly stopped being smothered by Monterey Jack? Basically, where would America be without the big cheese? But isn't it time we all put cheese in perspective?

I've lost count of the people I've talked with who have looked at me with longing and torment in their eyes as they said, "I love cheese but I gave it up," or "but cheese is BAD, isn't it?"

The good news for cheese lovers is that cheese does have nutritional attributes. It's a complete protein, it's a great source of calcium (200 mg per ounce) and other vitamins and minerals. But the bad news is that cheese is a high-fat animal product. Not only is it high in fat (usually around 73 percent of calories from fat), but a large portion of that fat is saturated. Then there's the issue of cholesterol. One ounce has about 28 milligrams of cholesterol.

Like many things, though, Americans seem to have exaggerated this whole cheese concept. Where else in the world do they take cheese strips (already having about 73 percent of calories from fat), deep fry them and call them appetizers? Where else do they offer "extra cheese" as an added topping on pizza? And how often at a party have you resisted saying, "Excuse me, sir, but would you like some cracker with your cheese?"

So, take it from a veteran cheese lover. We don't have to cut the big cheese out of our lives forever in order to eat a low-fat diet. We just have to start putting it into perspective. We can do this by following the "Say Cheese" Guidelines:

#1. *Don't eat cheese all alone.* I'm talking to those of you, and you know who you are, who open the refrigerator and automatically cut off a good-sized chunk of cheese and call it a "snack," or those of you who, when grating cheese for a recipe, end up saving about half of it from the grater by rescuing it into your mouth!

What "eating a low-fat diet" means is eating "meals" that are low in fat (making sure the percentage of calories from fat for the meal is less than 30 percent). So, theoretically, you can still eat high-fat items, such as butter and cheese, as long as the total meal stays under 30 percent of calories from fat. Which brings us to the next guidelines.

#2. *Only add cheese to low-fat foods—not other already high-fat foods.* This way the percentage of calories from fat for the meal has a chance of staying low overall. In other words, don't add cheese to something already high in fat, and don't add something already high in fat to cheese. The meal isn't big enough for both of them.

Sorry, but this puts the "cheeseburger" on the bad list, because the burger part is already contributing quite a bit of fat to the meal. And you can forget about your quiche recipe, because it already had tons of eggs, which are 55 percent calories from fat themselves. Adding lots of Swiss cheese won't help your fat content, not to mention the crust. This also means not topping your pizza with pepperoni or sausage, which would only add more fat. Try vegetables, onions, and mushrooms as your topping.

What we CAN add cheese to is our dear and faithful friends, the complex carbohydrates. If we follow guideline #3, we can add (in a low-fat way) cheese to our baked potato, our bagel, our pinto beans, and our pizza crust (if we don't overdo it), and still eat a low-fat meal.

#3. *Use less cheese.* Keep amounts of cheese more like a "sprinkle." (For this you'll need to pull out your grater.) Avoid slabs or slices. For example, if you add a tablespoon of Parmesan cheese to 1 1/2 cups of broccoli, it will have about 24 percent of calories from fat (and only 75 calories total). One cup of pasta noodles with 1/8 cup of grated cheddar cheese has only 20 calories from fat, 14 milligrams of cholesterol, and only 225 calories total.

A slice of cheese pizza (1/8 of a 14-inch pizza) has about 230 calories, 32 percent from fat, and 25 milligrams of cholesterol. You can add 1/8 cup of grated cheddar to your baked potato (21 percent calories from fat), an ounce of part-skim mozzarella to your bagel (22 percent calories from fat), or 1/8 cup of grated Monterey Jack (at most) to your refried beans (32 percent calories from fat).

#4. *Try to use lower fat cheeses as much as possible.* It really does make a difference. Adding an ounce of Monterey Jack will add 105 calories, 73 percent of which are from fat, and 26 milligrams of cholesterol. An ounce of part-skim mozzarella (and there are cheeses out now that are even lower in fat than this) adds about 78 calories, 55 percent from fat, and 18 milligrams of cholesterol. By the way, a tablespoon of Parmesan cheese adds only 23 calories, 60 percent from fat, 4 milligrams of cholesterol, and 94 milligrams of sodium.

As long as you "do" pretty much what these guidelines say, you can probably "say cheese" more often than you thought you could.

Just Say Yes to Lean Meats
Starting with Beef

In order to have a low-fat diet, do we need to "just say no" to beef? Absolutely not! We should, instead, start saying "yes" to the six leanest cuts beef has to offer.

All six cuts, when trimmed of their visible fat, have less than 42 percent of their calories from fat. This means when served with grains, vegetables, and other low-fat dishes, these cuts CAN be part of a low-fat diet:

(Per 1-ounce, cooked portion, already trimmed of visible fat)

- **Top Round,** 54 calories, 30.5 percent from fat, 1.8 grams of fat, 24 milligrams of cholesterol (sometimes called London Broil)

- **Eye Round Steak,** 52 calories, 32 percent from fat, 1.8 grams fat, 24 milligrams cholesterol

- **Round Tip, Sirloin Tip,** 54 calories, 36 percent from fat, 2.1 grams of fat, 23 milligrams cholesterol

- **Top Sirloin Steak,** 59 calories, 40 percent from fat, 2.5 grams of fat, 22 milligrams cholesterol (includes New York steak and strip steak cuts)

- **Tenderloin,** 58 calories, 42 percent from fat, 2.7 grams of fat, 24 milligrams cholesterol

Do you trim the visible fat from your meat BEFORE it hits the grill or pan? If so, you're slicing off slightly more calories, fat, and cholesterol than the person who waits to trim off the fat until it hits the plate. Besides bringing only the leanest cuts home with you and trimming off all visible fat before you cook it, there are two other steps you can take to keep meat part of the new low-fat way of eating:

- Cook the meat without fats or fatty sauces. Try grilling, broiling, roasting, or simmering slices in wine or chicken broth. In other words, once you've "cut the visible fat" try to avoid adding any fat back.

- This step might not be too popular with the bigger beef eaters, but it's an important one. Keep your servings to 3 ounces of cooked beef (4 ounces raw weight). That's about the size of a large chicken breast or the palm of your hand.

Does this take the fun out of eating meat? I hope not. To be perfectly honest, I think meat has never tasted better. You might think I'm a slightly biased consumer, but now when I think of sirloin, I picture it simmering in red wine with onions and garlic—instead of olive oil or butter.

Here are some tips for cooking lower fat cuts:

- To prevent dryness, do not over cook.
- Use slow, moist cooking methods, such as braising and stewing.
- Prevent natural juices from escaping. Avoid pricking or searing steaks while cooking.
- Salting meat before cooking tends to delay browning and draws out moisture.
- Marinate meats overnight when possible to increase tenderness. Marinades that include an acid ingredient, such as wine, vinegar, or lemon juice, will help break down some of the protein, making the meat more tender.

Think Lean

Have you ever wondered which red meat cuts have less fat than most? The following cuts have approximately 50 percent less fat (in grams) than the higher fat red meat cuts.

Each of the following cuts has:

- no more than 8 grams of fat per 3-ounce cooked portion (trimmed of all visible fat)

  AND
- no more than 80 milligrams of cholesterol

Beef:

Top round (London broil)

162 calories, 5.3 gms fat, 72 mg cholesterol

Eye of round

155 calories, 5.5 gms fat, 59 mg cholesterol

Round tip (sirloin tip, tip steak, or tip roast)

162 calories, 6.4 gms fat, 69 mg cholesterol

Sirloin (top sirloin steak)

177 calories, 7.4 gms fat, 76 mg cholesterol

Top loin (New York steak, strip steak)

172 calories, 7.6 gms fat, 65 mg cholesterol

Tenderloin (Filet Mignon, Chateaubriand)

174 calories, 7.9 gms fat, 72 mg cholesterol)

Pork:

Tenderloin

141 calories, 4.1 gms fat, 79 mg cholesterol

Lamb:

Leg shank portion

153 calories, 5.7 gms fat, 74 mg cholesterol

Leg, sirloin portion

174 calories, 7.8 gms fat, 78 mg cholesterol

Certain meats have, by themselves, less than 30 percent of calories from fat. This would also include most of the fish department, but first, let's list the low-fat meats, namely poultry light meat.

These cuts must contain:

• no more than 25 percent of calories from fat

AND

• no more than 90 milligrams of cholesterol per 3-ounce cooked serving.

Skinless chicken breast

141 calories, 69 mg cholesterol, 19 percent calories from fat

Skinless turkey breast

132 calories, 62 mg cholesterol, 18 percent calories from fat

Fish Hits the Big Time

One of my favorite less visible, less mobilized food councils has finally made the big time . . . or maybe I should say "prime time." The National Fish and Seafood Promotional Council must have recently gotten their advertising bucks together because they're hitting television prime time with some straightforward words about fish.

"Eat fish twice a week" is their main message to faithful television watchers everywhere, and a powerful message it is. Let's face it, most people aren't eating that much fish. In fact, most people probably weren't aware that this seemingly large amount of fish was recommended. And the ones who did already know are getting a friendly reminder.

Opting for fish as a source of protein instead of higher fat meat cuts or whole-milk dairy products, once in a while, will likely reduce the amount of saturated fat we eat. Of the 40 some odd items sold at a typical fish counter, there usually are at least 10 that have less than 10 percent of their calories from fat.

Read this list of some common fish and see if you hear any of your favorites. These are your lowest fat choices when it comes to finding fish.

Fish with 12% or less calories from fat

Alaska king crab	Blue & Dungeness crab
Octopus	Northern lobster
Pacific red snapper	Perch
Abalone	Grouper
Cod	Haddock
Bay scallops	Clams
Atlantic pollock	Lemon or Flounder sole
Yellow fin tuna	

Fish with 13% to 20% of calories from fat

Whiting	Monkfish
Sea bass	

I fully realize a certain class of fish, shellfish, has become notorious for being horribly "high in cholesterol." Besides squid, topping the high cholesterol fish charts with around 140 milligrams of cholesterol per 3 cooked ounces, shrimp comes in second with about 92 milligrams. Other popular shellfish selections, such as scallops (28 mg), oysters (46 mg), crab (35 to 65 mg), and lobster (57 mg), have reasonably less amounts of cholesterol per 3 cooked ounces.

How does shrimp's 92 milligrams of cholesterol compare with the leanest cut of beef? Three ounces of cooked top round, trimmed of visible fat, has about 72 mg of cholesterol. Surprised? Remember, the latest health guidelines for cholesterol in food recommend eating less than 300 milligrams a day. There's no reason why 3 ounces of shrimp (not fried, I hope) can't fit into that grand total every now and then.

Salvaging Your Favorite Recipes

Those of us who like to cook have favorite recipes we pull out from time to time. They're the torn ones with all the stains. Those of us who don't cook usually have at least a few dishes we're quite willing to beg people to make for us. And we certainly aren't emotionally prepared to lose these "favorites" to the health cause. However, chances are these "favorite recipes" aren't going to make the cut-offs in terms of fat content.

Since when did anybody "die for" broiled fish, pasta and steamed vegetables, or chicken stew? It's the oven baked lasagna, bacon quiches, and fettucini Alfredos of this world most of us consider our "favorites." And believe it or not, we CAN save most of these from the fat firing line by making some (hopefully not too painful) ingredient substitutions.

There are three ways to cut the fat in a recipe:

Way #1. Reduce the amount of fat called for. If the fat ingredient is a necessary part of the final product, then you may not be able to totally eliminate it. (Oil in pesto sauce is an example.) But you can usually DECREASE the amount added.

Way #2. Remove the fat ingredient entirely. Ask yourself whether the fatty ingredient is there primarily for appearance or out of habit or tradition (such as butter on cooked vegetables or whipped cream on strawberries).

Way #3. Use something else (lower in fat) instead. Is the ingredient there for flavor or texture? Can you get almost the same effect by adding another, lower fat item, such as low-fat yogurt to top your enchilada instead of sour cream or light mayonnaise instead of regular mayo in your tuna salad?

Now, try to have an open mind: This might mean using Egg Beaters egg substitute in your quiche (or mixing 6 egg whites or so with only 2 egg yolks), adding low-fat milk instead of cream and half the butter to your fettucini Alfredo, or mixing up a low-fat mushroom gravy for your stroganoff. Here are some suggestions. You can cut this guide out and stick it in your recipe box. Hopefully, in a few years, it too will be torn and stained.

Tip #1. **Instead of butter, shortening, or some margarines, USE**

- Butter Buds (a powder that looks like melted margarine once you add water) can be used to replace at least half the butter in many recipes, except to fry or sauté.

- A sprinkle or two of naturally flavored butter sprinkles (such as Molly McButter) over foods you might usually add butter or sour cream to.

- Margarine (where the first ingredient listed is a liquid vegetable oil). But remember, you're still replacing one fat with another, so add less if you can.

- Some or all of the butter, margarine, or oil in recipes can be replaced by another liquid that will add moisture. It all depends on the type of recipe as to how much fat can be replaced and by what (wine, fruit juice, chicken broth, etc.)

Tip #2. **Instead of baking chocolate (1 oz.) USE**

- 3 tablespoons cocoa plus 1 tablespoon oil

Instead of hot chocolate mixes, USE

- Hot cocoa mix made from:

1 cup nonfat dry milk powder

1/3 cup unsweetened cocoa powder

3 tablespoons sugar

(Mix ingredients and store in an airtight container.) To use, put 2 heaping teaspoons of mix into a cup and add hot water. Stir well.

Tip #3. **Instead of cheese, USE**

- Part-skim mozzarella and other reduced fat (lower calorie) cheeses. In most cases you can also use LESS cheese than the recipe calls for.

Tip #4. **Instead of ricotta cheese (whole milk) USE**

- Part-skim ricotta cheese or 1% fat cottage cheese, or a mixture of the two.

Tip #5. Instead of cream, USE

- Evaporated skim milk or regular low-fat milk. Add some nonfat dry milk if you need to thicken it. CAUTION! Nondairy creamers may have "no cholesterol" but most are just as high in percentage of calories from fat as cream.

Tip #6. Instead of cream cheese, USE

- Neufchatel cream cheese or Philadelphia Light or combine these with plain yogurt, part-skim ricotta, or low-fat cottage cheese.

Tip #7. Instead of creamy dressing or dip, USE

- Almost Fat-Free Creamy Dressing, made as follows:

  1 small envelope (1 oz.) ranch dressing powder
  (light if available)

  1 1/2 cups nonfat milk (or low-fat)

  1/2 cup nonfat plain yogurt (or low-fat)

  1 tablespoon "Lite" Miracle Whip
  (or reduced-calorie mayonnaise)

  Blend milk, yogurt, mayo, and powder together well. Keeps great in refrigerator about five days. Makes two cups of dressing.

Tip #8. Instead of eggs, USE

- Three eggs can be replaced by one egg beaten with three egg whites
- Egg Beaters (Fleischmann's) or egg substitute

Tip #9. Instead of gravy, USE

- Mushroom Gravy Mix:

  Mix 1 1/2 packets or cubes of low-sodium chicken broth (or beef) with 1 1/2 cups water. Add 3/4 cup raw sliced mushrooms and 1/3 cup diced onions. In a saucepan, simmer until the mushrooms are cooked and onions tender. In a separate pan, melt 1 tablespoon butter or margarine. Mix in 2 tablespoons flour. Add this to the mushroom mixture, stirring for a few minutes until the gravy thickens. Pour in 1/4 cup low-fat (or nonfat) milk and simmer, stirring for a few minutes longer.

Tip #10. Instead of mayonnaise, USE

- Plain yogurt
- Reduced-calorie types of mayonnaise
- Mock mayo: 1/2 cup reduced calorie mayo with 1/2 cup low-fat plain yogurt
- Low-fat cottage cheese, whipped up in a food processor or blender

Tip #11. Instead of whole milk, USE

- Nonfat or low-fat milk

Tip #12. Instead of oily vinaigrettes or marinades, USE

- For cold salads, try a reduced-calorie Italian dressing or Balsamic vinegar
- For marinades, try beer, wine, tomato puree, or low-sodium broths as your marinade base. Add garlic, spices, etc. as usual.

Tip #13. Instead of sour cream, USE

- Nonfat or low-fat plain yogurt (in sauces, add 2 tablespoons flour for each cup of yogurt so the sauce will thicken properly). For hot dishes, stir yogurt in just before serving, since high temperatures will cause it to curdle.
- Knudsen's Nice n' Light sour cream
- Formagg Sour Cream Style or other reduced fat "light" sour creams
- Substitute part-skim ricotta cheese or low-fat cottage cheese blended with buttermilk.

    CAUTION! Most imitation sour creams have just as much fat as regular sour cream.

Tip #14. Instead of sweeteners, USE

- In some cases, fruit and/or fruit juices or pureed fruits can be used for at least half the sugar called for.

Tip #15. Instead of some or all of the fat for stir-frying, simmering, or sautéing,

- Substitute low-sodium broths, wine, beer, or fruit juice.

Tip #16. Replaces some of the fat in certain recipes with

- Rum, whiskey, brandy, fruit juices and fruit purees (such as mashed bananas or applesauce), or buttermilk

NOTE: The alcohol in liquor evaporates during cooking.

Tip #17. Instead of bacon or sausage, USE

- Canadian-style bacon
- Louis Rich Turkey Breakfast Sausage
- The "half-the-fat" turkey bacon

Tip #18. Instead of ground beef, USE

- Ground sirloin (with less than 13 percent fat)
- Substitute ground turkey breast or ground chicken breast
- Healthy Choice 96% Fat Free ground beef

Making Recipe Changes

I know I may be repeating myself, but, hey folks, this is important. First, some practical lessons on how to lower the fat, then some sample recipes.

Lesson #1. Lite, Lighter, Lightest

As we speak, scads of ingredients that look, taste and act like the real full-fat versions, are sitting on supermarket shelves across America—willing and waiting to help you cut the fat in your favorite recipes.

The items listed here are the types of items you can use ounce for ounce, just like the regular products, and be assured of their success.

We're not substituting an entirely different ingredient for another here—we're simply using lower fat (or no fat) versions of the very same ingredient. Like using light or nonfat sour cream in place of the real thing in a dip or dressing, or using light or nonfat cream cheese to make cheesecake—like using lower fat Louis Rich Turkey Bacon, egg substitute and lower fat Swiss cheese in a Quiche Lorraine, or reduced calorie or fat-free mayonnaise in a pasta or potato salad.

Nothing too fancy folks, no big tricks, no secret substitutions. What could be more simple than adding low-fat milk, in place of cream or whole milk, to make a cream of broccoli soup or New England Clam Chowder. After all, both ingredients come from a cow, they're both white and liquid. Low-fat milk is just a little thinner, in its fat content and its consistency, that's all.

The past few years have been good to lower fat and fat-free products. Never before have so many "lighter" products been available to us. So many, in fact, it's hard to know what to use and in what proportions.

For many of these items it really comes down to personal preference. There are really three graduated steps; light, lighter, and lighest. Light means using the first level of reduced fat ingredients. Lighter generally means splitting the amount half and half with products listed in the light and lightest categories. And in the lightest list is where you'll find all the fat-free versions of common fatty ingredients.

A few people are destined for the lightest column because no matter how far you cut the fat, they're just not satisfied. They want to go all the way—they want to take it all out. But these people are few and far between. These are the people who, rather masochistically I might add, enjoy plopping plain nonfat yogurt on their potato, or are perfectly content drinking skim milk on a daily basis. These are the people who actually like the way the new fat-free cheeses and cream cheese taste. My husband and children are very happy to announce I'm not one of these people.

I'm personally most comfortable in the lighter column. I generally take it as far as I can while still producing a product very similar in taste and texture to the original high-fat recipe. Call me chicken, but my culinary conscience can't allow me to take away the aesthetic qualities that attracted us to these high-fat recipes to begin with. So find the place where you are most comfortable and take a look at the table below, listing lower fat ingredient options that are light, lighter, and lightest!

	Light	Lighter	Lightest
cream cheese	light cream cheese	1/2 light cream cheese 1/2 nonfat cream	nonfat cream cheese
cheese	reduced-fat cheeses	1/2 reduced fat cheese 1/2 fat-free cheese	fat-free cheese
sour cream	light sour cream	1/2 light sour cream 1/2 fat-free sour cream	fat-free sour cream
whipped cream	Cool Whip Light, Dream Whip or nondairy toppings	light whipped cream use less	1/2 whipped cream with 1/2 whipped eggwhites
milk	2% low-fat milk	1% low-fat milk	skim milk
evaporated milk	low-fat evaporated	1/2 low-fat evaporated 1/2 evaporated skim	evaporated skim milk
liquid cream	whole milk, low-fat milk or light whipping cream	evaporated low-fat milk	evaporated skim milk
eggs	1/2 eggs	fat-free egg	1/2 egg substitutes
mayonnaise	reduced-calorie "light"	1/2 reduced-calorie 1/2 nonfat mayonnaises	nonfat mayonnaises
bacon	use less of the real thing	Louis Rich Turkey Bacon	leave it out
sausage	Jimmy Dean light sausage	Louis Rich turkey breakfast sausage	leave it out
ricotta cheese	part-skim ricotta	low-fat ricotta cheese	fat-free ricotta
cottage cheese	2% low-fat cottage cheese	1% low-fat cottage cheese	fat-free cottage cheese
pastry crust	take the top crust away	take the top crust away, use a little less fat and a little more water when making the bottom crust	eliminate the crust or use Phyllo dough when possible, brush layers with margarine
creme fraiche	light sour cream	1/2 light sour cream 1/2 fat-free sour cream	fat-free sour cream

Lighten-Up Lesson #2: How Much Is Too Much?

The ultimate goal in this Lighten-Up Cooking Course is to reduce fat and calories, but without a detectable change in flavor, texture, and appearance. After all, we don't want to make the ultimate sacrifice—doing away with our enjoyment of food. Is this possible?

Definitely! But part of knowing how much is too much comes with experience and experimentation. Experimentation, however, can get a little time consuming, not to mention expensive.

And there is no simple answer because the amount of fat that can be taken out successfully, depends on each particular recipe. But you can get a better sense for how much is too much by asking yourself a few questions when you size-up each recipe:

Q #1—Is there a unique characteristic (like color, flavor, texture) that the fat or fatty ingredient is contributing to this recipe?

[Like whipped cream adding fluff in a mousse, or egg yolk adding color and texture in a Hollandaise sauce, or like the flakiness created by cutting butter or shortening into flour for a pastry crust or croissant.]

Q #2—Is there a lower fat version of the same ingredient that I can simply use instead?

[more information on this in Lesson #1]

Q #3—How much fat do I really need (or do I need it at all)?

[See "How Much Fat Do I Need" guidelines below]

Q #4—Can some of the fat be taken out and substituted with a nonfat ingredient?

Q #5—Can I add a little extra flavor using a nonfat or lowfat ingredient, to help compensate for the loss of flavor from the reduction or elimination of the fat or fatty ingredients?

Q #6—How much of the nice "extras" and fancy ingredients do I really need in this recipe? Can I get away with adding less or taking it out completely?

[In a chocolate chip cookie recipe, for example, you can often add about a third less chocolate chips and take out the nuts completely. You can also take out the extra chocolate chips and nuts that might be folded into a brownie batter.]

How Much Fat Do I Need?

General Guidelines

Remember, when you take fat out of a recipe, you often need to add another liquid ingredient (preferably one with low or no fat) to make up the difference in liquid volume and moistening power. So with the fat replacement rules in full force (see Lesson #3 for the specifics), you can often bring down the chief fat ingredient to the levels described below and still produce a food that looks and tastes like the original.

Muffins and nut breads

For a 12-muffin recipe, you can often bring down the oil, butter, or margarine to 2 tablespoons.

Homemade cakes and coffee cakes

Per cake, you can often bring down the butter, margarine, or oil to 1/4 to 1/3 cup.

Cake Mix

Since most cake mixes already contain about 4 grams of fat per serving, you don't need to add any of the oil called for on the box directions. Instead, add that amount of a nonfat liquid-type ingredient (like nonfat sour cream, applesauce, pineapple juice, flavored yogurt, evaporated skim milk, etc., depending on the flavor of the cake.)

Biscuits

The butter, margarine, or shortening can usually be reduced from 8 (1/2 cup) to 4 tablespoons for every 2 cups of flour. (But remember you must add 4 tablespoons of an appropriate fat replacement—like nonfat sour cream or nonfat cream cheese).

Pie Crust

The shortening, oil, butter, or margarine can usually be reduced to 3 tablespoons for every 1 cup of flour, with the added water increased to about 3 tablespoons for every 1 cup of flour.

Cookies

Generally you can cut the fat ingredient in half in most cookie recipes. (remember to add an appropriate fat replacement—like nonfat cream cheese)

White Sauces or Gravies

You can usually get away with cutting the butter down to about 1 teaspoon per serving of sauce. So if the sauce recipe make 4 servings, you can usually add about 4 teaspoons.

Cheese Sauce

Since the most vital flavor component in a cheese sauce is coming from the cheese, you can usually eliminate the added butter, or margarine entirely. Just make your thickening paste by mixing flour with a little bit of milk. Then whisk in more milk as called for in the recipe.

Tomato Sauce

Since the most vital flavor component in a red sauce is coming from the tomatoes, herbs and spices, very little or no olive oil needs to be added.

Marinades

The most important ingredient in the marinade is the liquid acid ingredient with tenderizing properties, not the melted butter or oil. So use the wine, beer, tomato juice, or vinegar as called for in the recipe (along with all the herbs, spices, and flavorings, such as onion powder or garlic), and reduce the oil or melted butter to a tablespoon per cup of marinade, or add none at all.

Vinaigrette Dressings

Because olive oil does add a characteristic flavor and mouth feel to a vinai-grette type dressing, you should probably add some olive oil. But the amount can be reduced to about 1 to 2 tablespoons of oil per 8 tablespoons of dressing. The amount of oil that you won't be adding should be replaced with a flavorful nonfat liquid (besides flavored vinegar, because you are already adding vinegar) like nonalcoholic wine or champagne, fruit juice, or fruit puree (such as raspberry or pear puree).

Frying and Sautéing

You don't really need to add any fat when frying or sautéing over the stove. Just add a nonfat liquid to serve the purpose fat would have.

Lesson #3 Fat Replacements in the Oven and on the Stove

When first attempting to modify those old (and new) high fat recipes, keep in mind fat was put there for a reason. When you think of fatty ingre-dients, you may first think about the flavors they add to recipes, but they also add other vital culinary characteristics like "moist crumb" in baking recipes, "good mouth feel", they even add texture to some foods. Fat also adds liquid measure to baking batters. On the stove, fat is a medium to con-duct heat and it keep foods moist while they cook.

You know the advertising slogan, "Everything tastes better with butter? Not only will I second that motion, but I would add a few more items to that list, like cream and cheese. But opting for the full amount of fat in a recipe is the easy way out. It's much more challenging to accomplish a wonder flavor without resorting to these old high-fat standbys. So when you reduce or nix the fat in a recipe, you have to REPLACE the lost amount of fat, preferably with something that will fulfill the same functions fat served in that recipe. This way the food is more likely to look, taste and feel like the original high-fat version.

There are two secrets to successfully cooking light: The first is knowing how much fat you can get away with taking out (refer back to Lesson #2 for more information) and the second is knowing what would make the very best fat replacement in that particular recipe.

The fat replacement has a tall order to fill. After all, you need to select something that will match many of the aesthetic and structural contributions of the original fat. For fat replacement suggestions in the oven or on the stove, see each special tip section below.

Fat Replacements in the Oven

One of the important cooking characteristics of fat in a baked batter or cookie dough is that it helps keep the crumb moist as it cooks in the oven. Unlike water, added fat doesn't blend chemically with the flour to make more of the bread, cake, or whatever you baking. Water also is a poor substitute for the moisture added by fat because water can be lost to evaporation during the baking, possibly drying the product.

So you are sometimes better off using a less-watery type of fat replacement which will retain most of its moisture during baking and tend not to blend with the flour towards a more bready result. For this reason I recommend nonfat and light sour cream as a fat replacement in many baked batters. In a rich cookie dough, I recommend nonfat or light cream cheese as a fat replacement (although in an oatmeal cookie, for some reason, nonfat or light sour cream seems to work well). These products have added gums and guars, which are soluble fibers and serve to hold onto the water nicely (on the supermarket shelf and in the oven).

In cake, muffin, or nut bread batters, flavored yogurts will usually serve you well as fat replacements, along with regular or concentrated fruit juices and fruit purees (like applesauce), low-fat milk or evaporated skim milk, or liquor or liqueurs.

When choosing a fat replacement, you should also factor in whether the fat replacement will impart the appropriate flavor to your baked item. If you don't want any other flavors competing with the flavors already in your batter (as in the case of cookies or chocolate brownies or cake), you are better off adding something like nonfat sour cream, nonfat cream cheese, vanilla yogurt, or evaporated skim milk, all of which will add a desirable creaminess without adding a strong flavor.

There are those times though, when you might welcome some additional flavor. When you reduce the oil in a carrot cake recipe, for example, you might want to use crushed pineapple in juice or applesauce as your fat replacement. These fruits will add an extra punch of fruity flavor while adding liquid to help compensate for the loss in oil. In a lemon or strawberry cake, you might select low or nonfat lemon or strawberry flavored yogurt as your fat replacement. In a yellow cake, you might want to replace half the missing fat with cream sherry to make a sherry cake.

One of the casualties of low-fat baking may be a shorter life-span for your cookie sheets and baking pans. But it usually is nothing that a good quality non-stick pan, a generous coat of non-stick spray, or a little elbow grease (and some hot soapy water) can't fix. You see, with normal high fat cookie batter, for example, the cookies are self-greasing because, while cooking, some of the fat melts out to create a nice greasy layer between the pan and the cookie. But when you bake lower fat cookies, you won't get this convenient but caloric layer of grease. Particles of the cookies are liable to stick to the the pan until they can be washed off.

To review, here's a list of possible fat replacements in the oven:

—nonfat or light cream cheese

—nonfat or light sour cream

—nonfat or low-fat flavored yogurts

—fruit juice and fruit purees

—liquor and liqueurs (sherry, grand marnier, whiskey, amaretto, etc..)

—evaporated skim milk

Fat Replacements on the Stove

There are basically three types of stove-top cooking methods that depend on the use of an indiscriminate amount of fat; sautéing, pan-frying and stir-frying. This fat seems to serve at least four purposes, most of which can be satisfied (to some extent) with an appropriate fat replacement. Fat adds a nonstick layer between the pan and the food; it serves as a medium to transfer heat from the pan to the food; and it keeps the food moist while it cooks. If olive oil, sesame or chili oil, or butter is called for, this cooking fat is also adding a distinctive flavor. In some cases, usually involving meat, fat also serves to help brown the food.

Most of the fat replacements listed below will perform all these functions, except maybe browning meat and adding the flavor of certain oils or butter. If either one of these functions is an absolute necessity, usually you can, at least, cut way back on the amount used. When stir-frying, for example, you can get away with using just a teaspoon of sesame oil or chili oil (for about 3 servings). Then when more oil is called for (usually a mild flavored vegetable oil), you can add a fat replacement cooking liquid instead (like low-sodium chicken broth, wine, beer, or fruit juice).

If a fatty alfredo sauce is more up your alley, you can get away with cutting the butter down to about 1 tablespoon for about 3 servings of sauce (and, of course, adding whole or lowfat milk, or evaporated skim milk instead of the cream). I find this adds just the right amount of butter flavor without going overboard on the fat.

When mixing up a gravy or stroganoff sauce, add nonfat sour cream instead of yogurt for a little added creaminess. Because of the gums and guars (soluble fibers) added to nonfat sour cream to keep them gelatinous, it won't separate out during heating like yogurt would.

Here's a list of possible fat replacements on the stove :

—low-sodium chicken, beef, or vegetable broth

—wine

—regular or nonalcoholic beer

—other liquor like brandy, vermouth, etc.

—fruit juices

—garlic wine

—flavored vinegars (if this flavor would be complimentary)

—plain old water

—low-fat milk or evaporated skim milk

—nonfat sour cream (especially to add creaminess to a gravy or sauce)

There is one use for fat that cannot be replaced with the aforementioned fat replacements—creating a crispy crust by frying something coated with a thick batter, flour, or crumb mixture, or wrapped in a thin layer of Chinese noodle (like with wontons or egg rolls) or phyllo dough. If you cook this in a watery liquid, the crust will become mushy and soggy, not brown and crispy as desired. In these cases, it might be preferable to oven-fry. This is where you take your crumb-coated or noodle-wrapped food and bake it on a lightly greased nonstick baking sheet. Baking it this way will not make the outside as bubbly as if you fried it in ample fat, but it will create a brown and crispy coating. A teaspoon or two of oil (not olive oil though, because it will breakdown and smoke at the higher temperatures) will usually suffice for a regular-sized baking sheet.

Flavor Without Fat

What's the number one reason people say they select (and eat) the foods they do? In a word—flavor. This is ONE aspect of food most Americans simply aren't willing to give up, even for such a good cause as health and longevity.

But you don't have to give up flavor for health—it isn't an either/or situation. Fat doesn't have the market cornered on flavor. Flavor comes in all shapes and sizes, all types of textures and colors. Consider for a moment, the likes of garlic, carmelized onions, balsamic vinegar, Grand Marnier, port wine, cinnamon, soy sauce, ginger, molasses, lemon juice, etc. Flavored vinegars can be used whenever you would use vinegar—particularly in salad dressing, marinades, and sauces. These all represent wonderful flavor possibilities, but none contribute fat.

Smoking is another way to add flavor. This particular cooking method perfumes its meat item with a unique, wonderful flavor, costing you little or no fat. When done correctly, smoked fish, chicken and turkey breasts, while very low in fat, can be extremely moist and tasty.

Why is flavor such a crucial concern in the Lightened-up kitchen? For every instance where a flavorful ingredient contains little or no fat, there are flavorful items full of fat (butter, cream, sharp cheddar, bacon, sausage, olive oil, chocolate, and the like). Many of our favorite recipes rely on these very fat sources for their distinctive flavors.

So when you reduce or remove these fatty ingredients, the truth is, you lose some of the flavor too. That's why when you take some or all of the fat out, you often need to compensate for the loss in flavors by adding new, complimentary flavors that don't come with fat. I tend to group these unappreciated, underutilized fat-free flavorings into 7 categories:

Liquor & Liqueurs	Flavored Extracts	Vegetables	Fruits	Herbs & Spices
Grand marnier	almond	ginger root	lemon	basil
Amaretto	mint	onions	lemon peel	dill
Vermouth	lemon	garlic	orange	tarragon
Sherry	rum	shallots	orange peel	oregano
Wine	vanilla	zest (peel)	limes	cumin
Beer	coconut			coriander
Creme de menthe	orange			fresh ground pepper
	liquid smoke			

Other Liquids
low-sodium soy sauce
flavored vinegars

High Flavored Sweeteners
molasses
brown sugar
maple syrup
concentrated fruit juices

❖ Sample Recipes ❖

Eggplant Parmesan

Original:

1 eggplant (about 1 to 1 1/2 pounds)

2 eggs, lightly beaten

1 cup Italian-style bread crumbs

9 Tbsp. olive oil

1 clove garlic, minced

1 can (28 oz.) crushed tomatoes

2 tsp. oregano

1/2 cup grated Parmesan cheese

8 oz. mozzarella cheese, shredded

Modified:

1 eggplant (about 1 to 1 1/2 pounds)

1 egg, 1 egg white, beaten with 2 Tbsp. water (reduced by 1 yolk)

1 cup cracker meal or white flour (lower in fat than bread crumbs)

1 1/2 recipe of "15 Minute Spaghetti" as follows:

9 oz. tomato paste, 21 oz. Italian-style stewed tomato, 7.25 oz. sliced bottled mushrooms, and seasonings

2 cups cooked pasta (use ziti macaroni or fettucini style). This adds carbohydrates to the recipe.

1 1/2 cups grated part-skim mozzarella cheese (about 7 oz.) (Lower in fat).

6 Tbsp. grated Parmesan cheese (reduced by 2 tablespoons)

NOTE: No oil is needed, since eggplant is broiled instead of fried.

Cut off stem and bottom of the eggplant, then slice off the lengthwise ends of the eggplant to eliminate tough skin. Cut the eggplant lengthwise into 1-centimeter-thick slices (usually makes about 10 slices). Coat each slice in egg mixture then in cracker crumbs. Place slices on a non-stick cookie sheet and broil each side at medium-high heat for about 3 minutes. Watch carefully so it doesn't burn.

Line a 9 by 9-inch baking pan with half the eggplant slices. Top with half the sauce, then half the mozzarella and 2 tablespoons of Parmesan. Now add the pasta evenly. Top with the rest of the eggplant, then the sauce and cheese. Bake for 15 minutes in a preheated 375° oven. Makes 6 servings.

Nutritional Analysis Per Serving (modified recipe):
Calories, 340; Fiber, 5 gm.; Cholesterol, 68 mg.; Sodium, 590 mg, Percent of calories from: Protein, 24%; Carbohydrate, 53%; Fat, 23%; In other eggplant Parmesan recipes, about 60 percent of calories are usually from fat!

The Art of Healthful Baking

Phase I

Contrary to what my friends think, I was NOT born a nutritionist. According to a certain third-grade document entitled "What I Want to Be When I Grow Up," I wanted to become a "baker."

Perhaps I was impressed by the hypnotic smell of bread baking, or maybe it was the taste of whipped cream—I just don't remember. But the point is, something else must have impressed me somewhere between third grade and college. Instead of writing about the "Joys of Baking with Lots of Fat," here I am writing about "The Art of Healthful Baking."

To be a "healthful baker," you have to be committed to minimizing the two favorite baking ingredients: fats (butter, lard, vegetable shortening, oil, take your pick, they're all "fat") and eggs (specifically egg yolks). Remember, eggs have more than 50 percent of their calories from fat, so we're minimizing them not only because they're high in cholesterol, but because they are a fatty ingredient. And while we're at it, it's not a bad idea to minimize sugars (white, brown, powdered, or honey) and salt (sodium chloride) when possible.

By making a few ingredient adjustments, we can transform your favorite baking recipe into a more healthful food. You may have to get used to the color, light brown, if half the flour you add is whole wheat. And if you lower the fat and sugar, the crumb may not be quite as smooth and moist or the taste as sweet—depending on how low you go. In many cases, you can cut the fat and sugar in half without anyone noticing, including you!

Experiment using the guidelines below until you've lowered fat and sugar as far as you can while still maintaining the taste that keeps you making that recipe again and again.

Yeast Breads

These recipes aren't usually the fat and sugar culprits. Only a small amount of sugar (about 2 tablespoons) is added to help the dough rise and brown the crust. Shortening (fat) is not an essential ingredient but is added to give flavor and make the crumb tender. Try to keep it down to 1 tablespoon per loaf.

Quick Breads (nut breads, muffins, cornbread, biscuits)

With quick breads, added fat can be lowered in several ways:

- Use nonfat milk instead of whole milk. (Nonfat milk contains all the protein and other nutrients without the fat and extra calories.)
- If eggs are used, keep to a maximum of one per recipe.
- Try not to add too many nuts (only about 1/4 to 1/3 cup per loaf).
- Keep the fat ingredient (shortening, butter, oil, etc.) to a minimum (about 2 to 3 tablespoons per recipe). With biscuits, you can cut the added fat by a third or a half, but you may then need to use a little more nonfat milk to help mix in the extra flour.
- Sugar can usually be reduced to about 2 to 3 tablespoons per recipe.

Cake Squares, (spice and carrot cake, coffee cake, pound and fruit cake)

In cooking circles, these desserts are informally called "butter cakes," and for a very good reason!

You can reduce fat in several ways:

- The first suggestion will probably be the toughest to follow: Strip the frosting off the cake. Frosting is made of only fat and sugar. So the only way to reduce them is to decrease or eliminate the frosting altogether. (You'll be amazed how well carrot or spice cake stands on its own.)

- Depending on the recipe, sometimes you may be able to cut the fat in half. (A minimum of about 1/4 to 1/3 cup of added fat usually is essential.)

- If 3 eggs are called for, use 2 instead.

- Sugar may be reduced to a minimum of about 1/3 cup.

- To lighten the cake's texture, you can beat egg whites separately and fold them into the batter toward the end.

Very Important Messages

- Remember, every time you take fat OUT of a recipe, you need to add the same amount of fat-free liquid back in to keep it moist and tasty. Fruit juices work well with muffin-type batters and some cake recipes, while liquor (rum, whiskey, brandy, sherry, etc.) works well in others. If you cut oil from 6 tablespoons to 2 tablespoons, you'll need to add at least 4 tablespoons of fruit juice back.

- When substituting whole-wheat for white flour, use 7/8 cup instead of 1 cup.

Pies and Pastries

The sugar in the pie filling can be cut in two, at least. Sometimes only one-fourth of the sugar listed in the recipe is really necessary!

To lower fat:

- Pie crust is made of fat and flour. A quick way to decrease fat is to take the top crust off your pie. Instead, sprinkle toasted oatmeal or graham cracker crumbs on top or cover with a meringue. Also, you could just cover the pie with foil when baking (to prevent loss of moisture). Then serve it with ice milk on top.
- Don't dab any butter inside the pie or on the crust.

Following these guidelines, you can take an ordinary peach pie, at 584 calories per serving and 41 percent of those calories from fat, and turn it into 311 calories per serving with 34 percent of calories from fat.

Let's take a look at how I changed one of my favorite recipes:

Carrot Cake (Without Frosting)

Original ingredients:

3 cups carrots

2 cups flour

1 cup sugar

1 1/2 cups oil

1/2 cup unsweetened coconut

3 eggs

1/2 cup walnuts

1 tsp cinnamon

2 tsp baking powder

2 tsp baking soda

1 tsp salt

This recipe contains:

570 calories per serving, 3.5 grams fiber, 80 milligrams of cholesterol, and 63 percent of the calories from fat.

Modified recipe:

3 cups carrots

1 cup whole-wheat flour

1 cup white flour

1/2 cup sugar

1/3 cup oil

1 cup orange juice

8 oz canned pineapple in juice

1/2 cup unsweetened coconut (optional)

1 egg and 2 egg whites

1/3 cup walnuts

1 tsp cinnamon

2 tsp baking powder

1 tsp baking soda*

*No salt is needed because baking soda and powder already contain sodium.

This recipe contains:

215 calories per serving, 2.7 grams fiber, 22 milligrams of cholesterol, and 36 percent of the calories are from fat.

Phase II

Something New, Lesson 1

All that salt the recipes tell you to add? Don't listen to them. It's more than optional; it's totally unnecessary. Only in yeast breads is a moderate amount needed to help control the yeast activity. You're going to get plenty of sodium in your baking powder (247 mg per teaspoon) and baking soda (821 mg per teaspoon). These are not optional unless you like your cakes and muffins flat as a board.

Something New, Lesson 2.

Ration only one egg yolk per recipe. That's usually all you need to keep your batter smooth and blended. Remember, every last drop of fat and cholesterol is neatly tucked away in the yolk of the egg. So if the recipe normally calls for 2 eggs, use 1 egg and 1 or 2 egg whites.

Something New, Lesson 3.

Try to get used to a light brown crumb and the nutty taste of whole-wheat flour. Just by using 1 cup of whole-wheat flour and 1 cup of white instead of 2 cups of white flour, you double the amount of dietary fiber (15 grams instead of 7). And, as a bonus, you get a veritable vitamin bonanza! Indeed, you can double the amount of vitamin B6, folacin, pantothenic acid, copper, phosphorus, potassium, selenium, and zinc and get one and a half times more vitamin E and calcium and two and a half times more magnesium just by using half whole-wheat flour in your recipe.

The Something Old, Lesson 4.

Now, for the sake of review, here's a lesson on something old. (It's starting to sound like someone is getting married.) In most baking recipes, you can automatically cut the fat and sugar in half without anyone noticing. Just remember to make up the difference in liquid volume lost by adding a fruit juice. For example, if you cut the amount of added oil in a muffin recipe from 1/2 cup to 1 tablespoon, you will need to add about 6 tablespoons of orange or pineapple juice.

Chapter 7

What's the Big "Fat" Deal About Homemade Meals?

The First Meal of the Day —Break-fast.

Breakfast, the MOST important meal of the day? Well, that's debatable. (I place my vote for the mid-day lunch.) But for most of us, it's obviously the FIRST meal of the day anyway. What we choose to put into our bodies will, in essence, fuel half of our workday. Think about that next time you're feeding yourself before a big meeting!

Certainly, children seem to function better in school with breakfast in their stomachs. Recent clinical research on children suggests they have a definite decrease in problem-solving abilities on mornings when they skip breakfast. But, back to us adults who may not need to master times tables in the morning.

I have some clinical research results to cite for you, as well. This may sound a bit extreme, but it makes an interesting point. In a Midwestern study, overweight people who received their entire allotment of the day's calories at breakfast actually lost weight, while most of the people who took in all their calories at dinnertime gained weight instead.

Many of us tend to do the same breakfast day after day. So I would suggest we make sure whatever it is, it's low in fat. There's a huge difference, for example, between chewing on a croissant or Danish and fixing a bowl of hot oatmeal. And there's something to be said for washing your breakfast down with orange or grapefruit juice instead of creamed and sugared coffee each morning.

Avoiding the buttery croissant or jelly-filled donut and Danish is probably a predictable suggestion. But what about those gourmet muffins or freshly baked bagels that come with at least a one- to two-ounce slab of cream cheese in the middle? Well, I hate to burst your health-muffin bubble, but most commercial muffin recipes (yes, even the bran types) usually have at least 40 percent of their calories from fat, with up to 400 calories each and 30 to 60 milligrams of cholesterol—mainly from eggs added to the batter. A bagel, by the way, with half an ounce of Neufchatel cream cheese has about 200 calories, 21 percent from fat, and 11 milligrams of cholesterol.

And now a few words on cereal. Somehow hot cereals have gotten the reputation of being too time-consuming to cook. Not necessarily true. Most are even microwaveable or about 5 minutes from start to finish to cook over the stove. This is hardly time intensive. It will take you at least 5 minutes in line at that bakery of yours. Of course, we need to make sure we're not adding too much fat to our cereal. We can add fruits for flavor instead of butter. Dried fruits, such as raisins, or dried apricots or fresh fruits, such as banana coins or peach slices, can be added. Even cooked fruit, such as applesauce or apricots with cinnamon, will make a tasty cereal topping.

We can pour non- or low-fat milk over our cereal instead of "whole milk" where almost half the calories come from fat. Non- or low-fat milk is great for cooking those instant oatmeals in too, instead of water. When we add 1 cup of skim milk to 1 1/2 cups of cooked oatmeal in place of 2% low-fat milk, the percentage of calories from fat falls from 24 percent to 11 percent.

On weekends, we're in a different breakfast mode altogether, aren't we? Suddenly we start imagining Belgian waffles decorated with berries and whipped cream, three-egg omelettes, or a stack of pancakes. Pancakes and waffles are workable, but that three-egg omelette is a fat-laden no-no, anyway you top it. The basic ham and cheese omelette without sour cream has about 725 calories—70 percent from fat, and 850 milligrams of cholesterol. See what I mean?

So what do Americans do to these horribly high-fat, cholesterol-rich breakfast entrees? We eat them with more fatty foods, such as bacon, sausage, or hash browns on the side. You might ask, "All right, Elaine, what DO we do?" If you eat eggs occasionally, try lightening them up by adding a few egg whites to one whole egg. (This is for two people.) Beat in some nonfat milk and maybe one or two tablespoons of flour or low-fat cottage cheese (to thicken it up) and your eggy entree is MUCH lower in calories and cholesterol and has around 26 percent of its calories from fat. You can even fill your new fluffy omelette with nonfat items (tomatoes, onions, mushrooms, salsa, plain yogurt, etc.).

In the '90s, eggs may have a brighter future. Or, I should probably say, egg whites, because all the fat and cholesterol, as you know, is in the yolk. You might want to give some of those already blended "new-age" eggs out of a carton a try. The brand lowest in fat, Fleischman's Egg Beaters, is mostly egg white blended with some natural yellow coloring. It can be used in your quiches and puddings as well as for the typical scrambled egg or omelette. Granted it isn't the same, but in most cases it'll do just as well.

Certain high fat foods, which won't remain nameless, that we usually eat with our eggs drive an already dangerously high-fat breakfast completely over the cholesterol cliff. Three small strips of bacon add 120 calories, 9 grams of fat, and 16 milligrams of cholesterol, while 3 pork sausage links add 790 calories, 65 grams of fat, and 140 milligrams of cholesterol.

But in the 90's even this aspect of our egg-consuming behavior is improving. As a former BLT lover, I've been searching for a lower-fat bacon look-alike for years. I'm happy to announce one has finally arrived! Turkey Selects from Armour came out with a Turkey Breakfast Strip that has 66 percent less fat than bacon. Turkey Breakfast Links are also available.

Even the United States Department of Agriculture recently cut the egg yolk some slack. Due to refined feeding practices and more sophisticated chemical lab tests, the department recalculated the average large egg yolk as having 213 milligrams of cholesterol, quite a step down from the 274 milligrams previously estimated. But don't start counting your eggs before they hatch. . . 213 milligrams is still high compared to the health recommendations that limit daily dietary cholesterol to less than 300 milligrams.

Looks like the day could be saved after all for the All-American egg, even in this age of low-fat living and egg-yolk rationing.

Breakfast on the Run

Morning after morning, most of us rush, rush, rush around the house to get ourselves out the door on time, just to sit on a freeway somewhere in the typical urban commute. Well, if we're going to be inching along bumper to bumper, we might as well have a nice relaxing breakfast while we're at it.

Having your breakfast on the run does have a couple of shortcomings that we might as well admit to right away. You can't read the newspaper while you eat your breakfast anymore (unless you're in the passenger's seat), and you can't have gooey, messy breakfasts anymore (you know, the ones where you really do need to use a fork and knife).

And you'll need to stock your car (now doubling as a breakfast nook on wheels) with a few supplies. Keep your glove compartment well stocked with napkins. Get a beverage holder for your dashboard or center console if you don't already have one. And if you tend to stain your clothing with even the "hard-to-spill" foods, you might want to keep a small towel in the back that you can drape over your clothes while you leisurely eat and drink your breakfast. Of course, we aren't talking about toting the usual "fast" breakfast foods, such as a cheese Danish and coffee or an Egg McMuffin. Here are five low-fat ideas, one for each day of the work week. If you keep things on schedule, you can even remind yourself what day it is. "If it's muffins, this must be Tuesday," for example.

#1. Make Your Own Frozen Waffles

You can pop them directly from the freezer into the toaster, wrap them in a paper towel, grab some juice or fresh fruit, and you're out the door. You can use the basic instructions for buttermilk waffle batter, but to keep them low-fat, use about 2 cups of flour (1/2 whole wheat if you want), 1 1/3 teaspoons baking powder, 1 tablespoon sugar, 1 egg yolk, 2 egg whites, 1 3/4 cup buttermilk, and at the most, 2 tablespoons oil. If you absolutely need to grease your waffle iron, try using the Weight Watchers or PAM sprays. These waffles come out to about 236 calories each (this recipe makes six waffles) that are 15 percent calories from protein, 60 percent carbohydrate, and 25 percent from fat (using 2 tablespoons of oil). Cholesterol is 45 milligrams and sodium, 150 milligrams per large waffle. After cooking, break the waffles into toastable-sized squares, place a servings worth in a plastic bag, and store in the freezer.

#2. Leftovers Fit for Breakfast

For those craving the atypical breakfast, even cold pizza will do. One slice of cheese or vegetarian pizza, 1/8 of a 14-inch pizza, has about 230 calories, 30 milligrams of cholesterol, and 580 milligrams of sodium. From 30 to 35 percent of calories are from fat, 20 percent from protein, and up to 50 percent from carbohydrate. The less cheese, the better. Because this breakfast is a little high in fat, make sure to drink some fruit juice or eat a piece of fresh fruit with it.

#3. The Way Yogurt Lovers Eat Their Cereal

Figure out a steady place in your car to set your bowl down. Then find a plain nonfat or low-fat flavored yogurt. Most flavored yogurts go heavy on the sugar, so watch that, too. If a flavored yogurt has around 150 calories per 8-ounce serving (such as Weight Watchers brand), it usually is the lower sugar type. Assuming you've already been using a low-fat, high-fiber cereal, you're ready to add about a cup of your cereal to your cup of yogurt. For smaller eaters, cut down to 3/4 to 1/2 cup of each.

#4. Bagel Delights

Keep your already-split bagels in the freezer. Then in the morning you just need to break them apart and toss them in the toaster. While they're toasting you can get the mystery ingredient ready. If you feel like a toasted onion and cheese bagel, you can slice your cheese while your onion bagel is toasting. If it's more of a bagel and cream cheese morning, get your 1/2 ounce of Neufchatel cheese (or Philadelphia Light) ready to spread.

• A toasted onion bagel with an ounce of cheese has 265 calories, 28 milligrams of cholesterol, 500 milligrams of sodium, 21 percent of calories from protein, 49 percent from carbohydrate, 30 percent from fat, and 215 milligrams of calcium. Using a lower fat cheese will help bring the fat down further.

- A bagel with 1/2 ounce of Neufchatel or light cream cheese has about 200 calories, 11 milligrams cholesterol, 310 milligrams sodium, 16 percent of calories from protein, 64 percent from carbohydrate, and 20 percent from fat.

  If you add 2 tablespoons of Smucker's low-sugar preserves to the above, it's 250 calories, 13 percent from protein, 70 percent from carbohydrate, and 17 percent from fat.

- An English muffin (or bagel) with 1 tablespoon of peanut butter will be about 245 calories, 0 milligrams of cholesterol, 255 milligrams sodium (if you use the unsalted type), 15 percent of calories from protein, 55 percent from carbohydrate, and 30 percent from fat.

#5. My Favorite Muffins

Think about it: You can take muffins camping, to a picnic, or impress your colleagues and bring a batch to your next early morning meeting. But there is one tiny problem—that three letter word again: FAT.

The muffins you buy in your friendly neighborhood bakery (even the bran types) are usually pretty packed with grease—40 percent or more of calories from fat. This is about the same as a biscuit, and some come close to looking more like a Danish (with 50 percent of calories from fat) than a muffin.

The newer, fancy muffin mixes (Bran & Honey-Nut or Cinnamon Swirl, for example) have vegetable shortening (a saturated fat) listed as the third ingredient. The second and fourth ingredients are sugar in the Cinnamon Swirl case. The Swirl will come out to about 32 percent of calories from fat, but only because the sugar content is so high it brings down the percent of total calories from fat.

What is the answer to the over-fat and sugar-laden muffin? Just three little words. Make your own! It's easier than you think. Make a batch on Sunday night, have a couple for breakfast on Monday, and freeze the rest in individual serving bags. Come Wednesday or Friday morning, you just take one or two out of the freezer and pop them into a microwave or toaster oven for a couple of minutes. To make low-fat muffins, follow the "Art of Healthful Baking Guidelines" on page 165.

I also need to qualify that some bakery muffins are better in the fat department than others. So it's possible your favorite bakery muffin is just fine. How can you tell? Well, you can't really tell for sure, but here's one quick clue. Try the muffin grease spot test:

Cut your muffin in half. Take one of the halves and press the just-cut side to a brown paper bag. (You can see the grease spots better if the bag is brown.) Or use a paper towel or napkin, if that's what is handy. Then look for grease spots on the towel or napkin.

It doesn't take a trained eye to be able to tell the difference between a grease spot and a water or juice spot. If you're not sure, touch it with your fingers. You can almost always feel the difference.

To get you started on your merry low-fat muffin way, there are two quick and easy recipes for my favorite muffins in the recipe section in the next chapter.

Don't Forget Your Fruit
(or Fruit Juice)

A cup of orange, grapefruit, or pineapple juice totals 100 to 140 calories. They're all mostly carbohydrate calories. This helps round off your breakfast on the run. I like making a big enough fruit salad to last a few days. Then in the morning all I have to do is scoop some out into a portable container and off to work I go. Fresh fruit makes a great mid-morning snack.

Now for one last quick breakfast tip. Keep some of the microwaveable instant oatmeal envelopes (the less sweetened ones) in your desk drawer at work. Then all you need to do is buy some non- or low-fat milk at the cafeteria, pop the cereal and milk into the microwave for two minutes, and you've got yourself a breakfast—or an afternoon snack, for that matter.

Packing a Low-Fat Lunch Box for Your Child

It doesn't matter whether your child is going to school or playing at home. That daily question continues: "What should I fix for lunch?"

It's not a simple question either. You want it to be healthful; you want it to meet their nutrition and growth needs. But most important of all, you want them to like it because chances are they won't eat it otherwise. Which brings me to the subject of VARIETY. It's not only the spice of life, it's the spice of the lunch box, too. Back in grade school, I remember bag lunch after bag lunch filled with Nilla wafers, carrot sticks, and those little boxes of raisins. I'm just now (15 some odd years later) getting to the point where I can eat raisins and carrot sticks again. I still can't face Nilla wafers.

The bottom line to a bag lunch is, does your child actually eat it? This makes it imperative your child is included in the "what's for lunch" discussion. This doesn't mean you magically become a short-order cook an hour each day. But try to consider your child's likes and dislikes as best you can. Some kids will gladly share these with you again and again. With other kids, you might have to do some probing. Try asking which type of bread they like best. What are their favorite sandwiches?

Only after my poor horrified mother found two weeks worth of decaying, uneaten sandwiches under my bed did she come to the understanding I hated chewy sticky white bread getting stuck in my teeth and to the roof of my mouth. So here's another question to ask. Do you like your bread toasted or plain?

What are the essential ingredients to a child's healthful bag lunch? It should include some fresh fruit or fruit canned in juice, and some vegetables. Vegetables can be sliced and added to the sandwich or cut up into sticks or coins, washed well, and put into a bag. (Otherwise they dry up by lunchtime.) If the lunch doesn't already include an ounce and a half of cheese on a slice of pizza or in the sandwich, then you might want to add a small carton of non- or low-fat milk or some yogurt. Or give your child the money to buy that at school.

Dessert? I must admit I definitely remember looking forward to eating the chocolate covering off and unrolling the Ho Ho every day. The "dessert" or something special concept isn't all that bad. It's the "what" we consider (or what we train our children to consider) dessert or special that gets us into trouble. There are healthier cookies out there and great recipes for muffins and nut breads that can certainly double as dessert. Many are included in the next chapter.

The main feature of your child's bag lunch can obviously be the standard sandwich, but it can also be, your child's preference permitting, something on the order of leftover lasagna, chili with cornbread, or colorful vegetarian pizza slices. Which standard sandwiches should be more standard than others? Believe it or not, the esteemed peanut butter and jelly sandwich can make this healthful sandwich list—with a few minor adjustments. Here are a few of the possibilities:

Peanut Butter and Jelly Sandwich

2 slices whole-wheat bread

2 tablespoons peanut butter

2 tablespoons Smucker's Low-Sugar spread

Nutritional Analysis:

410 calories, 7 grams fiber, 510 mg sodium, no cholesterol, 15 percent calories from protein, 50 percent from carbohydrate, 35 percent from fat

CLT
(Cheese, Lettuce and Tomato)
Sandwich

1 1/2 oz. part-skim cheese

Half a tomato, sliced

2 slices whole-wheat bread

Several leaves of dark green lettuce

Mustard to taste (analyzed with 1/2 teaspoon)

Nutritional analysis:

300 calories, 4 1/2 grams fiber, 600 mg sodium, 27 mg cholesterol, 25 percent of calories from protein, 48 percent from carbohydrate, 27 percent from fat. (The fat content jumps to 37 percent if regular cheese is used.)

Meatball
Surprise Sandwich

10 small meatballs (or 4 medium-sized meatballs) from the "Italian-Style Hamburger or Meatball" recipe found in the next chapter (page 231)

1 French or sourdough roll

1 to 2 tablespoons catsup or tomato sauce

1 tablespoon grated Parmesan cheese (that's the surprise)

Nutritional Analysis:

425 calories, 55 mg cholesterol, 780 mg sodium, 26 percent of calories from protein, 52 percent from carbohydrate, 22 percent from fat

Turkey

2 slices whole grain bread

2 1/2 ounces cooked turkey breast, sliced thin (You can buy the whole turkey breasts cooked in the packaged meat section of the supermarket.)

A few leaves of dark green lettuce

Half a tomato, sliced

Mustard to taste or 1 tablespoon cranberry sauce

Nutritional Analysis:

295 calories, 5 grams fiber, 50 milligrams cholesterol, 420 mg sodium, 38 percent of calories from protein, 48 percent from carbohydrate, 14 percent from fat

A Few Fruit Ideas

Try orange or apple wedges, sliced bananas, pears, canned apricots (in juice), 100 percent pure orange, apple, or grapefruit juice.

Try mixing and matching the above, such as pineapple chunks with banana coins and raisins, or apple wedges with pears and cinnamon.

Some Cuttable Vegetables

Try cucumber, zucchini, carrot, and celery strips or sticks, cauliflower or broccoli florets, kohlrabi, carrot, cucumber or squash slices or coins, green or red pepper rings.

Adults Need Lunch, Too

Many of the same principles for your child's lunch box apply for you, too—the need for fruits and vegetables, choosing lower fat snacks and goodies. Perhaps your choice in sandwich might differ. There are a few fancy (low-fat) sandwich recipes for you in the recipe section in the next chapter. The lunch tips listed in the Deli Delights section in Chapter 5 also can be helpful at home.

But "lunch" certainly isn't synonymous with "sandwich." Warmed up chili or casseroles make great lunches from home. This doesn't take any extra time, either. All you need to do is plan for leftovers when you're making dinner. Then package individual portions directly into microwaveable storage containers. Keep one for tomorrow's lunch, then freeze the rest. I find people are far more willing to eat "leftovers" at lunch than at dinner two days in a row. Besides, if the recipe is considered delicious, then you and your family will even look forward to lunches.

When I eat out at a restaurant on a weeknight, I usually go so far as to eat half my meal and doggy bag the rest for tomorrow's lunch. You can order a couple of "a la carte" items in addition to your dinner selection, and tell the waiter or waitress to package them to go. And there you have it— your ready-made lunch for tomorrow.

Curious About Condiments?

I can show you how to make a low-fat hamburger patty, but all the trimmings are up to you. And don't underestimate the contribution that condiments can make towards the fat total of the meal. Some of them are definitely NOT benign "extras." Here's a list of the more popular condiments

1 Tablespoon	Calories	% Calories from fat	Sodium (mg)
Mustard	11	8%	188
Ketchup	16	6%	170
Chili sauce	16	trace	201
Cocktail sauce	20	trace	160
Sweet pickle relish	21	4%	197
Steak sauce	18	trace	149
Sweet & sour sauce	32	trace	320
Reduced-calorie mayonnaise	35-50	90%	115
Tartar sauce	75	96%	182
Mayonnaise	100	100%	78

Obviously, in terms of adding fat, mustard or ketchup is the better choice than mayonnaise to spread on your bread or bun. If mayo is a must, then opt for the reduced-calorie types (giving you half as much fat per tablespoon). And then just "wet the bread," don't smother it with the stuff.

In these tables and recipes we measure condiments in teaspoons and tablespoons, but when it comes to actually spreading, we're measuring in spoonfuls or a knife's worth. So get yourself (and your loved ones) very well acquainted with what a teaspoon or tablespoon really looks like. For most people, one tablespoon doesn't even begin to describe the amount of mayonnaise or tartar sauce they usually add.

CAUTION: Most sandwich shops use large plastic spatulas to spread their mayonnaise. I find the specifications "just barely wet the bread" are much more effective than "spread it light, will ya?" What that person thinks is "light" and what you think is "light" could be a tablespoon apart.

Life Beyond
the TV Dinner

We think we have to choose between making a laborious dinner from scratch and eating a frozen or fast food dinner. Fortunately, it isn't that simple. This myth lives on because all the recipes we ever come across in magazines and newspapers require at least 10 ingredients. (Many require an extra shopping trip because you certainly don't have half that stuff at home.) Also, many recipes require an hour of preparation time.

Let's face it. After a long day at work, we don't have an hour to give. The solution? New recipes to make at home that require a reasonable amount of preparation time. They say we all basically have 20 recipes we end up making over and over. So I'm asking you to incorporate some new ones (low in fat) into your 20 recipe repertoire AND to revise the rest using the guidelines listed in the beginning of this chapter. You might find some of your favorites have already been revised in the recipe section that follows, such as low-fat lasagna, macaroni and cheese, and tacos.

Don't be put off by the amount of time some of these recipes require in the oven. This is still FREE TIME for you—time you can use to ride your stationary bike, soak in the tub, read the newspaper, or play with your kids. The bottom line here is that it takes less time in the kitchen, right?

My two favorite quick and easy dinners are the "two P's": pasta and potatoes. I like to buy fresh pasta noodles (you can freeze pasta, too). And while it's boiling, you can get your low-fat sauce and vegetables ready. If I'm really in a hurry, I throw my vegetables in with the pasta and let them both boil. There are a couple of low-fat sauces in the recipe section, but you can also use Ragu Gardenstyle Spaghetti Sauce in a bottle, a reduced-calorie Italian dressing, or just toss a mixture of Parmesan cheese, black pepper, and natural flavored butter sprinkles, such as Molly McButter or Best O'Butter.

Once in a while I'll even spend a Saturday making homemade ravioli (my secret filling recipe is found in the next chapter: "Chicken, Basil, Baby Carrot Filling"). Then you freeze a dinner's worth in separate plastic storage bags. All that's required when you come home from work is to take a bag out of the freezer and boil some water. Homemade pasta in minutes!

For a quick potato dinner, you can pop your potatoes into the microwave until they're cooked throughout (5 to 10 minutes, depending on how many potatoes and your microwave). While they're cooking, start getting your filling and topping ready. Fill each potato with vegetables, such as onions, mushrooms, squash, etc., or lean meats such as leftover London broil or chicken breast. You can even open a can of water-packed tuna. Top the potato with Ragu Gardenstyle or other low-fat red sauces, a cheese sauce (see the next chapter for recipe), Parmesan or part-skim milk cheese.

These are just two examples. There are many more in the recipe section.

Here's another handy tip for you:

After making a batch of burritos or quesadillas, you always seem to have a couple of tortillas left. Because they will dry out quickly in their torn plastic bag, you go through the trouble of tucking them safely into a ziplock bag, only to find them a few weeks later in the back of your refrigerator, green with mold.

Well, hold that ziplock—because there is another lower-fat use for that flour tortilla. Thick, homestyle flour tortillas make a quick quiche crust. And they're much lower in fat and calories than the traditional pastry crust. Here are the directions for your tortilla quiche crust:

It usually takes exactly two 7 to 9-inch tortillas to cover a regular 9-inch pie pan. Just lightly grease your pie or quiche dish with diet margarine. Then press one of the tortillas into the pan so it is off center and up one side of the dish. Cut the second tortilla in half and piece the halves into the pan to fill the two spaces. If the tortillas need to be softened before they can be pressed into the pan, sprinkle some water on both sides, heat in a non-stick fry pan on low, flipping frequently, until they are pliable. Proceed with the rest of your quiche recipe. Bake as usual until tortilla crust is lightly brown and quiche is cooked throughout (about 40 minutes). A two-tortilla crust adds only about 250 calories and 6 grams of fat to the whole pie. Compare the differences:

	Pie Crust	Tortilla Crust
Preparation Time (1)	5 minutes	2 minutes
Calories per Pie	900	250
Fat grams per Pie	60	about 6

Chapter

Cooking Smart: Recipes for Lowering Fat

❖ Breads and Muffins ❖

Lemon Bread

2 cups flour

1 cup whole-wheat flour

4 tsp baking powder

3 Tbsp margarine or butter, softened

1 cup sugar

1 egg

3 egg whites

1 cup low-fat milk

finely grated peel of 2 lemons (2 tsp)

Glaze: Filtered juice of two lemons mixed with 2 Tbsp powdered sugar

Preheat oven to 350°. Mix together flours and baking powder. In separate bowl, cream the margarine with the sugar. Stir in egg and egg whites, lemon peel, and any pulp filtered from the lemon juice. Blend with flour mixture and pour into two nonstick sprayed loaf pans (9 x 5"). Bake until toothpick inserted near center comes out clean. (About 30 minutes. Don't over bake!) Brush hot loaves with lemon glaze. Makes 24 slices (12 per loaf).

Nutritional Analysis: Per slice

Calories 113, Fiber 1 gm, Cholesterol 15 mg, Sodium 70 mg, Percent of calories from: Protein 10%, Carbohydrate 75%, Fat 15%

Apricot Nut Bread

1 1/4 cup whole-wheat flour

1 cup white flour

1 tsp baking soda

1 tsp baking powder

1 tsp cream of tartar

1/2 tsp salt

2 eggs

1 1/2 cup orange juice

3 Tbsp oil

1/2 tsp vanilla extract

1/2 cup sugar

8 oz dried apricots, chopped

1/3 cup walnuts

Preheat oven to 350°. Lightly beat eggs with orange juice. Add oil, sugar, and vanilla. Mix dry ingredients. Add wet and dry mixtures together, not over mixing. Toss in apricot and walnut pieces. Bake for about 45 minutes. Makes 2 loaves, 10 servings per loaf.

Nutritional Analysis: Per serving
Calories 140, Fiber 3 gm, Cholesterol 26 mg, Sodium 116 mg, Percent of calories from: Protein 8%, Carbohydrate 67%, Fat 25%

Lemon Zucchini Bread

1 egg and 2 egg whites

1 cup sugar

1/4 cup oil

2 tsp vanilla

1/2 cup lemon yogurt (non- or low-fat)

2 tsp grated lemon peel

2 cups grated zucchini

2 cups flour (you can use 1/2 whole wheat and 1/2 white)

2 tsp ground cinnamon

2 tsp baking powder

1/4 tsp salt

1/2 cup chopped walnuts or pecans (optional)

Preheat oven to 350°. Lightly coat 2 standard loaf pans with non-stick spray. Mix dry ingredients together and set aside. In medium bowl, beat eggs until frothy (a minute or so) then beat in sugar, oil, vanilla, yogurt, and lemon peel. Stir in zucchini and dry ingredients. Add nuts if desired. Pour into two loaf pans. Bake for 45 minutes to 1 hour (until fork inserted in center comes out almost clean). Let bread cool 15 minutes before removing from pan. Makes 16 thick slices (8 per pan).

Nutritional Analysis: Per Slice
Calories 153, Fiber 1 gm, Cholesterol 17 mg, Sodium 80 mg, Percent of calories from: Protein 8%, Carbohydrate 69%, Fat 23%

Apple-Spice Bran Muffins

1/2 cup white flour
1/2 cup whole-wheat flour
1 cup wheat bran
2 tsp baking powder
1/2 tsp baking soda
1/4 tsp salt (optional)
1 tsp ground cinnamon
1/4 tsp ground nutmeg
1/8 tsp ground cloves
1/4 cup egg substitute (or 2 egg whites)
3/4 cup unsweetened applesauce
1/3 cup brown sugar
1/4 cup nonfat plain yogurt
1/2 tsp vanilla
1 Tbsp vegetable oil
1/2 cup raisins (optional)

Lightly grease muffin pan or use non-stick spray or paper baking cups. Stir flour, bran, baking powder, baking soda, salt, and spices together in medium bowl. In another bowl, combine egg substitute with applesauce, sugar, yogurt, vanilla, oil, and raisins. Add egg mixture all at once to the dry mixture. Stir just till moistened. Spoon batter into muffin cups filling each three-fourths full. Bake in 400° oven for 15 to 18 minutes (for regular-sized 2 1/2-inch muffins) or until done. Makes 10 muffins.

Nutritional Analysis: Per muffin (without raisins)
Calories 105, Fiber 3 gm, Cholesterol 0 mg, Sodium 118 mg, Percent of calories from: Protein 11%, Carbohydrate 75%, Fat 14% (1.7 gm)

Fruit and Bran Muffins

1 egg

1 cup low-fat milk

1 cup wheat bran

1/2 cup whole-wheat flour

1/2 cup white flour

14 cup honey

1 Tbsp baking powder

1/2 tsp salt (optional, but this recipe was analyzed with it)

1 tsp cinnamon

1 Pippin apple

3/4 cup crushed pineapple (do not drain)

2 Tbsp butter or margarine, melted

Preheat oven to 375°. Put the egg, milk, honey, butter, and bran in a mixing bowl and let stand for 5 minutes. Meanwhile, finely chop apple. Add the flours, baking powder, salt, cinnamon, apple, and pineapple. Stir until barely mixed. Spoon into muffin papers, filling each cup until almost full. Bake in the middle of the oven for about 20 minutes. Makes 8 muffins. They can be frozen and defrosted as needed.

Nutritional Analysis: Per Muffin
Calories 170, Fiber 4 gm, Cholesterol 44 mg, Sodium 285 mg, Percent of calories from: Protein 10%, Carbohydrate 67%, Fat 23%

Banana Health Nut Muffins

2 medium very ripe bananas

3 Tbsp butter or margarine, very soft or melted

1/2 cup pineapple juice

1/2 cup sugar

1 egg, 1 egg white

1/2 cup walnut pieces

1 cup whole-wheat flour

1 cup white flour

1/4 cup wheat germ

1 tsp baking powder

1/4 tsp ground cloves or 1/2 tsp cinnamon

Preheat oven to 400°. Mash bananas thoroughly in mixing bowl. Add the next four ingredients and blend until smooth, using electric mixer if possible. Mix in nuts. In another bowl, mix dry ingredients until well blended. Gradually add dry mixture to liquid mixture, mixing well with electric mixer. Spoon batter into Teflon muffin pan or paper baking cups. Bake until lightly brown, about 20 minutes. Makes 12 muffins.

Nutritional Analysis: Per Muffin

Calories 210, Fiber 2.45 gm, Cholesterol 30 mg, Sodium 80 mg, Percent of calories from: Protein 9%, Carbohydrate 62%, Fat 29%

Blueberry Oat Bran Muffins

2 1/4 cups oat bran (a mixture of 1/2 rolled oats and 1/2 oat bran may be used)

1/4 cup chopped nuts

1/4 cup raisins

2 tsp baking powder

1/4 cup honey

1 egg with 2 egg whites, beaten

1 Tbsp vegetable oil

2/3 cup blueberries, raspberries, or chopped apricots (frozen berries can be used)

1/2 tsp cinnamon

Preheat oven to 425°. In a large bowl, combine first four ingredients. Add remaining ingredients. Mix until dry ingredients are moistened. Fill Teflon muffin pans (or use paper liners) until almost full. Bake 15 minutes or until golden brown. Makes 12 muffins.

Nutritional Analysis: Per Muffin

Calories 150, Fiber 2.5 gm, Cholesterol 22 mg, Sodium 60 mg, Percent of calories from: Protein 15%, Carbohydrate 59%, Fat 26%

Low-fat Garlic Bread

8 oz part-skim ricotta cheese

2 Tbsp butter or margarine, melted

1/4 cup grated Parmesan cheese

1 Tbsp Best O'Butter (or Molly McButter)

3 cloves garlic, finely minced

1 1/2 lb French or sourdough bread

Preheat oven to 400°. Blend first five ingredients together well. Cut bread loaves into two halves each. Spread the garlic mixture on evenly. Bake for 5 to 7 minutes. (Broil for a short time at the end, if you prefer.) Slice into separate pieces. Makes 15 dinner servings.

Nutritional Analysis: Per Serving

Calories 168, Cholesterol 10 mg, Sodium 325 mg, Percent of calories from: Protein 15%, Carbohydrate 66%, Fat 19%

Easy Cheesy Biscuits

1 cup whole-wheat flour

1 cup white flour

4 tsp baking powder

1 cup nonfat milk

1/2 cup chopped onion

3 Tbsp butter or margarine

2.5 oz part-skim cheddar cheese (about 1/2 cup), grated

2 tsp herb of choice (I like to use Italian seasonings)

Preheat oven to 350°. Simmer onions in margarine for about 5 minutes. Meanwhile, mix dry ingredients. Then mix everything together, stirring just until blended. Spoon into Teflon-coated muffin pan. Makes about 12 biscuits. Bake until lightly brown (about 10 to 12 minutes).

Nutritional Analysis: Per Biscuit

Calories 125, Fiber 1.5 gm, Cholesterol 4 mg, Sodium 155 mg, Percent of calories from: Protein 15%, Carbohydrate 55%, Fat 30%

Lighten-Up Classic Egg Dishes

I seem to have rediscovered the nutritionally infamous egg lately. Perhaps because for the past year I have been able to serve them, guilt-free, to my almost 2-year-old daughter. But most of us, without infants, rediscover eggs and the classic egg dishes during that annual occasion that pairs bunnies with eggs and chocolate with both—Easter.

So in honor of bunny day and all subsequent lunches and brunches, I've lightened-up four classic egg dishes—from the common omelette to the elegant Eggs Benedict.

Omelette Tips

- For an unusually fluffy omelette, that will puff up in the pan, some of the white and yolks may be beaten separately before being folded together. See the recipe on the next page for what I've found is an ideal proportion of egg substitute and fresh egg yolks and whipped egg whites. Air is incorporated into the whites during the beating. So that the trapped air does not escape, blend whites with the yolk/egg substitute mixture immediately and make omelettes without delay.

- Fresh herbs like marjoram, parsley or a mixture with chervil, chives or tarragon, bring fragrance to an omelette without adding any fat or calories. Dried marjoram or oregano are good aromatic substitutes.

- Diced butter is usually beaten into the egg batter (with MORE butter used in the pan during cooking). You can completely cut out the butter in the batter and seriously reduce the butter in the pan to about 1/2 teaspoon per omelette (or you can even use nonstick spray in a nonstick pan if you'd rather).

- Preparation tips:
  - Heat pan thoroughly before adding eggs
  - Cook over medium-high heat to create firm exteriors with soft interiors
  - Prepare in a heavy omelette or crepe pan

Fluffy Omelette for Two

1/2 cup egg substitute

2 eggs, separated

Herbs and seasonings as desired

Low-fat fillings as desired

Blend egg substitute and egg yolks in medium bowl and set aside. Whip egg whites until stiff. Fold carefully into egg yolk mixture. Heat omelette pan or small nonstick fry pan. Generously coat with nonstick spray (or use 1/2 tsp margarine or butter). Spread half of mixture in pan. Heat until top looks firm (about 2 minutes). Fill with desired fillings or sprinkle with desired seasonings and fold. Remove to serving plate. Repeat with remaining egg mixture. Makes 2 fluffy omelettes. Serve with low-fat accompaniments to bring down the percentage of calories from fat for the meal.

Nutritional Analysis: per serving

Calories 105, Cholesterol 210 mg, Sodium 163 mg, Percent of calories from: Protein 50%, Carbohydrate 7%, Fat 43% (5 grams fat)

Matty's Scrambled Eggs Au Gratin

To lighten-up this wonderful egg dish, I reduced the butter and used low-fat milk to make the white sauce. Then I used half real eggs and half low-fat egg substitute (which is mostly egg whites) for the scrambled egg part. I grated Cracker Barrel Light Sharp Cheddar and switched to Louis Rich Turkey Bacon. This dish turned out so well, even my egg-detesting husband ate it.

1 Tbsp butter or margarine

3 Tbsp flour

1 1/2 cups 1% milk

1/4 tsp salt

1/4 tsp pepper

2 1/2 cups sliced mushrooms

3 Tbsp vermouth or sherry

3 eggs

3/4 cup low-fat egg substitute

1/4 cup 1% milk

6 strips Louis Rich Turkey Bacon, cooked and crumbled

4 ounces reduced fat sharp cheddar cheese, grated

Preheat oven to 325°. Melt 1 Tbsp butter in small saucepan. Add 3 Tbsp (from the 1 1/2 cups) of milk. Blend in flour until smooth. Slowly whisk in the remaining milk. Simmer, stirring constantly, until thickened. Season with salt and pepper. Set aside. In medium fry pan, simmer mushrooms in vermouth until cooked (cover pan). Remove with slotted spoon. Beat eggs and egg substitute with milk. Coat fry pan with nonstick spray (or melt 1 tsp butter to coat bottom). Pour in eggs, stirring over medium heat until tender. In 2-quart casserole dish, combine turkey bacon, cheese, mushrooms, eggs and white sauce. Stir to blend. Bake for 25 to 30 minutes. Serves 6. Serve with low-fat accompaniments to bring down the percentage of calories from fat for the meal.

Nutritional Analysis per serving

Calories 204, Fiber 0.5 gm, Cholesterol 127 mg, Sodium 528 mg, Percent of calories from: Protein 36%, Carbohydrate 20%, Fat 44% (10 gm fat). NOTE: The original recipe contained 317 Calories, 25 gm fat, and 268 mg cholesterol per serving

Eggs Benedict

To lighten-up the hollandaise sauce (which, for all intents and purposes, is basically egg yolk and butter), I eliminated one of the egg yolks and most of the butter. I added some flour and low-fat milk to make up the difference and cut the salt in half. And because the sauce still contained 2 egg yolks and lemon juice, the distinctive color, texture and flavor remained almost the same. I bypassed the step of buttering the toasted English muffins altogether. I also used a very lean ham and sizzled it in a nonstick fry pan coated with nonstick spray. I poached the eggs in a couple tablespoons of brandy, for a little added flavor. Personally, I find it easy to split each egg in two and top each prepared muffin with 1/2 of a poached egg—but how far you want to take this lower fat/lower cholesterol thing is obviously up to you! When I tested this recipe out on notorious Eggs Benedict lovers, they couldn't even tell the difference.

Hollandaise Sauce:

   2 egg yolks

   1/4 tsp salt

   1/8 tsp pepper

   2 Tbsp lemon juice

   2 Tbsp orange juice

   3 Tbsp butter or margarine

   2 Tbsp flour

   3/4 cup 1% low-fat milk

      (add more milk if a thinner consistency is desired)

8 eggs, poached
16 thin slices lean smoked ham (about 5 or 6 oz)
4 English muffins, halved and toasted
Paprika
Fresh parsley sprigs

For sauce, place egg yolks, salt, pepper, lemon and orange juice in food processor or blender. Blend at top speed for 2 seconds. In nonstick saucepan over medium heat, melt 3 Tbsp butter. Blend in flour until smooth. Quickly whisk in milk, a little at a time. Whisk in egg yolk mixture and continue to heat, stirring constantly until nicely thickened. Trim the ham to be slightly larger than muffins. Sizzle each two slices of ham together in a nonstick fry pan that has been lightly coated with nonstick spray. After turning ham over, add Madeira if desired. Lay two slices of ham on each muffin half. Top with egg and cover with warmed hollandaise sauce. Sprinkle with paprika and garnish with parsley. Serves 8. Serve with low-fat accompaniments to bring down the percentage of calories from fat for the meal.

Nutritional Analysis per serving
Calories 237, Fiber 1 gm, Cholesterol 288 mg, Sodium 596 mg, Percent of calories from: Protein 24%, Carbohydrate 32%, Fat 44% (11.5 gm fat). Each serving of the original recipe contains: 480 calories, 42.5 gm fat, 411 mg cholesterol! **NOTE:** To reduce cholesterol and fat further, use only 4 poached eggs and place half an egg on each muffin. Each serving will now contain 200 calories, 9 gm fat, and 182 mg cholesterol.

Less Deviled Eggs

6 whole eggs

2 Tbsp 1% low-fat (or nonfat) cottage cheese, whipped in food processor
to remove lumps

1 Tbsp reduced-calorie mayonnaise

1 Tbsp fat-free or light sour cream

1 1/2 tsp Dijon mustard

Pepper and seasonings to taste

Lemon juice to taste (about 1/2 tsp)

Paprika

Gently boil 6 eggs until hard boiled. Let cool. Remove shells and cut each
egg in half lengthwise. Remove yolks. Toss three of the yolks. In food
processor, blend remaining yolks with whipped cottage cheese, mustard, fat-
free sour cream and reduced-calorie mayo until smooth and creamy. Add in
lemon juice, pepper and/or selected seasonings to taste. Spoon yolk mixture
into pastry tube or metal cake decorating press. Squeeze yolk mixture decora-
tively into 12 egg white halves. Lightly dust with paprika if desired. Makes
12 halves.

Nutritional Analysis: per half

Calories 27, Cholesterol 53 mg, Sodium 46 mg, Percent of calories from:
Protein 41%, Carbohydrate 6%, Fat 53% (1.5 gm). **NOTE:** Regular deviled
eggs contain around 58 calories, 5 gm of fat, (75% calories from fat) and
108 mg cholesterol, per half an egg. (Values vary slightly depending on the
recipe.)

❖ Soups and Salads ❖

In Search of a Great (Low-Cal) Salad Dressing

Has it been so long since many of us made our salad dressings fresh that we've forgotten how great they taste? Have we slowly become so desensitized to the artificial and processed flavors of most reduced-calorie and nonfat bottled salad dressings that we don't even notice anymore how different they really taste from the regular types? Compared to the regular versions, in my experience, most of these lower calorie dressings leave a lot to be desired.

The fact that so many of us have just come to accept their taste deficiencies became quite apparent when, during a taste test of various fat-free and reduced-calorie ranch dressings, my husband exclaimed, "they all taste like plastic to me!" Suddenly, as if a deep fog had lifted from my taste buds, it occurred to me—that's why salads eaten in restaurants taste so good—fresh, regular calorie dressings!

I would rather drizzle 1 tablespoon of the real thing over my salad greens than 1/4 cup of the fat-free stuff. That's one option, of course. The other is to improve the flavor of reduced-fat/calorie salad dressings by making them fresh at home. This was quite a revelation for someone like me who grew up with an assortment of bottled dressings in the refrigerator at all times.

Why might these bottled low-cal dressings taste so plastic and unsavory? The answer might lie in their long list of ingredients. The sheer quantity of ingredients is mind boggling. The bottle of low-cal ranch sitting in my refrigerator listed exactly 28 items. When you make them fresh at home you might mix 4 or 5 ingredients together, tops. When you make them fresh at home you don't need items like propylene glycol alginate (added for consistency), calcium disodium EDTA and TBHQ (added to "protect the flavors"), or polysorbate 60. Could the essence of plastic be coming from these ingredients? I wonder.

So with a little experimentation here and a little substitution there, I've come up with quick, homemade (lower fat) recipes for the four most popular flavors in salad dressing: Thousand Island, Ranch, Blue Cheese, and Italian. Sure it takes a few more minutes to whip these dressings up fresh, but the improvement in flavor is well worth its "wait" in gold.

Bleu Cheese

Bleu cheese itself is so full of flavor, you don't need that much of it to make a great, sharp tasting dressing. Because of the potent flavor of bleu cheese, it isn't necessary to use the full-fat sour creams or mayonnaises. Just let the flavor of the bleu cheese come through and add reduced-calorie mayo and nonfat sour cream instead.

2 oz. bleu cheese
1/4 cup reduced-calorie mayonnaise
Juice from 1 lemon
1 tsp Dijon mustard
1/4 cup nonfat sour cream

Whip all ingredients in a food processor until blended. Make about 3/4 cup.

Nutritional Analysis: per 2 tablespoons
Calories 56, Cholesterol 12 mg, Sodium 161 mg, Percent of calories from: Protein 21%, Carbohydrate 19%, Fat 64% (4 gm fat). Fat and calories can be reduced even further by using nonfat mayonnaise.

Thousand Island Dressing

1/4 cup reduced-calorie mayonnaise

1/4 cup fat-free mayonnaise

2 tbsp catsup

1-2 tablespoons minced stuffed olives or dill pickles

1 tbsp minced onion

2 tsp parsley flakes

Optional items:

1/2 tbsp chopped green pepper

1/2 hard-cooked egg, chopped

Combine the above ingredients and serve over salad greens. Makes about 3/4 cup of dressing.

Nutritional Analysis: per 2 tablespoons of dressing

Calories 54, Fat 3.4 gm, Cholesterol 3 mg, Sodium 300 mg, Percent of calories from: Protein 1%, Carbohydrate 44%, Fat 55%

Vinaigrette Dressing

1/8 tsp salt (or to taste)

1/4 tsp pepper

1/4 tsp garlic powder

1/4 tsp dry mustard

1 Tbsp olive oil

1 Tbsp lemon juice

Combine the above ingredients and beat well with a wire whisk until smooth.

Add:

3 Tbsp apple juice, wine or beer

Whisk well and add:

1 to 2 Tbsp Balsamic vinegar

1 Tbsp olive oil

1 Tbsp red wine vinegar

Whisk well and refrigerate. Shake well before using. Makes about 9 table-spoons of dressing.

Nutritional Analysis: per 2 tablespoons of dressing

Calories 60, Fat 6 gm, Cholesterol 0, Sodium 58 mg, Percent of calories from: Protein 0, Carbohydrate 14%, Fat 86%

Potato Cheese Soup

6 medium-large red potatoes, cooked

3 cups nonfat milk

6 oz sharp cheddar cheese, grated

1 1/2 cups chopped white onion

1 Tbsp fresh parsley, finely chopped

1/4 tsp pepper (or to taste)

1/2 tsp sweet basil leaves, dried

Paprika (optional)

Mash potatoes and onions together until smooth (as if you're making mashed potatoes) or use a food processor. There might be a few potato chunks, but that's fine. Add potatoes to a large soup kettle and mix in the milk and spices, except paprika. On medium heat, let simmer for about 8 minutes, stirring frequently. Then mix in the grated cheese. Let simmer about 8 minutes longer. Serve in bowls. Lightly sprinkle paprika on top if you like a little pizzazz or color. Makes about 6 servings. Freezes well, too.

Nutritional Analysis: Per Serving

Calories 275, Fiber 5 gm, Cholesterol 30 mg, Sodium 247 mg, Percent of calories from: Protein 21%, Carbohydrate 48%, Fat 31%, (When served with bread, the percent from fat will decrease a bit.)

Autumn Medley Stew

2 (15-ounce) cans stewed tomatoes

1 yellow onion, cut into strips

2 or 3 medium carrots, sliced into coins

1 green pepper, coarsely chopped

2 potatoes, raw, diced

3 chicken half breasts

2 cups water (with 2 packets low-sodium chicken broth mix, optional)

4 cups cooked rice

1/2 tsp black pepper

1 tsp rosemary

1 tsp Italian seasoning

4 cloves garlic, crushed

In a large soup kettle, simmer chicken breasts in 2 cups of water (or chicken broth). Add onion to chicken as it simmers. While it's cooking, slice the other vegetables. When chicken is cooked throughout, remove and set aside. Add tomatoes, potatoes, carrots, peppers, and spices to onion and broth mixture. Continue to simmer. Break chicken into chunks, de-bone, and add to stew. Simmer 30 minutes or until carrots and potatoes are tender. Add rice and simmer 10 minutes longer. Makes about 8 servings.

Nutritional Analysis: Per Serving
Calories 214, Fiber 4.5 gm, Cholesterol 22 mg, Sodium 215 mg, Percent of calories from: Protein 24%, Carbohydrate 70%, Fat 6%

Less Fat Potato Salad

4 lbs white potatoes (or red), microwaved or baked until done, then diced

1 green pepper, finely chopped

1 red pepper, finely chopped

1 cup chopped green onion (use white and part of green)

1 cup thinly sliced celery

1 1/2 cup bread and butter pickles, diced

3 hard boiled eggs, cooled then chopped

Dressing:

8 oz low-fat cottage cheese (use 1% milkfat if available)

3/4 cup reduced-calorie mayonnaise

2 Tbsp Dijon mustard

1/2 to 1 tsp dillweed

2 Tbsp parsley flakes (crushed in hand as you add)

1 tsp black pepper

Toss the first seven ingredients in a large bowl. Using a food processor or blender, whip the cottage cheese until it looks smooth. Then add the mayo, mustard, and spices, and whip again until well blended. Stir dressing into potato salad mixture. If you tend to like less "other stuff" in your potato salad, reduce the pepper, celery, and pickles by half. Makes 15 servings, at least!

Nutritional Analysis: Per Serving
Calories 190, Fiber 4.5 gm, Cholesterol 55 mg (with eggs), Sodium 290 mg
Percent of calories from: Protein 14%, Carbohydrate 67%, Fat 19%

Garden Rice Salad

1 1/2 cups cooked brown rice (or wild rice blend), cooled
1 1/4 cups chopped tomatoes
3/4 cup lightly cooked peas (microwave frozen peas on high for 2 minutes)
1/4 cup finely chopped green onions (remove half of green top)
1/4 cup pine nuts
    (broil for a minute or so to brown, if possible)

Dressing:

2 Tbsp lemon juice
1 tsp walnut oil (or olive oil)
1/4 tsp black pepper
1/8 tsp garlic powder
1/2 tsp oregano
1/2 tsp sweet basil

Toss the first five ingredients together in a medium bowl. In a small bowl, mix the dressing ingredients. Stir the dressing well while pouring evenly over the rice mixture. Toss together and chill in refrigerator until ready to serve. Makes 4 servings.

Nutritional Analysis: Per Serving
Calories 153, Fiber 6 gm, Cholesterol 0 mg, Sodium 12 mg, Percent of calories from: Protein 13%, Carbohydrate 66%, Fat 21%

Macaroni Salad

12 oz uncooked macaroni noodles

1 1/2 cups red bell pepper, finely chopped

6 green onions

3/4 cup green pepper, chopped

1 1/2 cup celery, sliced

1 3/4 cup bread and butter pickles (finely chopped)

1 lemon, squeezed on top of salad and tossed (optional)

Dressing

1 1/2 cup low-fat cottage cheese (1% milkfat)

1/3 cup reduced-calorie mayonnaise

1 Tbsp mustard

1 tsp pepper

1 tsp crushed dried basil leaves

1 tsp dill, dried

Cook macaroni as directed on package, drain, and cool. While noodles are cooling, chop and prepare the remaining ingredients. Add the cottage cheese to a blender or food processor. Whip until smooth and creamy. Add the mayonnaise, mustard, and seasonings to the cottage cheese and mix by hand. When pasta cools, toss with remaining ingredients, add dressing, and blend. Serves 12.

Nutritional Analysis: Per serving
Calories 170, Fiber 2.5 gm, Cholesterol 3 mg, Sodium 335 mg, Percent of calories from: Protein 18%, Carbohydrate 71%, Fat 11%

Quick Tuna Salad

1 6.5-oz can water-packed tuna, drained
1 apple, diced
3 Tbsp reduced-calorie mayonnaise
2 cups shredded salad greens

Toss tuna, apple, and mayonnaise together. Serve over salad greens (or on bread for a sandwich.) Makes 2 servings.

Nutritional Analysis: Per Serving (with salad greens)
Calories 230, Fiber 3 gm, Cholesterol 52 mg, Sodium 409 mg, Percent of calories from: Protein 44%, Carbohydrate 36%, Fat 20%

Creamy Fruit Salad

2 cups assorted fresh fruit (for example, 1 cup strawberries,
    1 sliced peach, 1 sliced banana)
1/2 cup lemon or vanilla low-fat yogurt
Dash cinnamon or nutmeg

Toss yogurt with fruit. Top with cinnamon. Makes 2 servings

Nutritional Analysis: Per Serving
Calories 142, Fiber 4 gm, Cholesterol 3 mg, Sodium 39 mg, Percent of calories from: Protein 10%, Carbohydrate 82%, Fat 8%

Sunshine Salad

4 cups fresh spinach

2 nectarines, sliced

1 cup fresh strawberries, halved

6 Tbsp reduced-calorie vinaigrette

1 Tbsp sunflower seeds, toasted

Toss first four ingredients together. Sprinkle sunflower seeds on top. makes 4 servings.

Nutritional Analysis: Per Serving

Calories 81, Fiber 4.4 gm, Cholesterol 0 mg, Sodium 220 mg, Percent of calories from: Protein 13%, Carbohydrate 62%, Fat 25%

Caesar Salad

5 Tbsp apple juice

1 tsp gelatin

1/4 tsp chopped garlic

2 Tbsp olive oil (or other)

1/4 tsp dry mustard

Juice from 1 lemon

4 anchovies drained and mashed into a paste

3 Tbsp wine vinegar

A few drops Worcestershire sauce

1/4 cup egg substitute

3 Tbsp Parmesan cheese

12 cups romaine lettuce pieces

3/4 cup croutons

In 1-cup measuring cup, sprinkle 1 teaspoon of gelatin over 2 tablespoons of the cold apple juice. Let stand 2 minutes. Microwave on HIGH for 30 seconds; stir thoroughly, then let stand 2 minutes or until gelatine is completely dissolved. In a food processor or blender, blend this mixture with remaining apple juice and the garlic, oil, mustard, lemon, anchovy paste, vinegar, Worcestershire sauce, egg substitute, and Parmesan cheese (or leave the cheese out and sprinkle over the dressed lettuce). Let stand 30 minutes or so. Toss with romaine lettuce and top each serving with about 2 tablespoons of croutons. Makes about 6 side servings.

Nutritional Analysis: per serving
Calories 108, Fiber 2 gm, Cholesterol 5 mg, Sodium 222 mg, Percent of calories from: Protein 20%, Carbohydrate 30%, Fat 50% (6 gm fat)

Ramen Cabbage Salad

2 Tbsp sliced almonds

2 Tbsp sesame seeds

10 oz shredded cabbage (about 6 cups), all green or red and green

3 green onions, finely chopped (white portion and half of green)

1 cup canned black beans, drained and rinsed

1 package Campbell's Low-Fat Chicken
   Flavor Ramen Noodle Soup

Dressing:

3 Tbsp honey

2 Tbsp apple juice

3 Tbsp rice vinegar

1/2 Tbsp sugar

1 Tbsp sesame oil

Toast sesame seeds and almonds separately by laying them in a single layer of a pan and broiling carefully until lightly brown. Set both aside. Put cabbage, almonds, sesame seeds, onions, and beans in serving bowl. Add Ramen noodles after crumbling them into small pieces with your hands. Mix dressing ingredients well with wire whisk. Drizzle over cabbage mixture and toss. (Make sure you mix dressing just before tossing with salad.) Makes 6 salad servings.

Nutrition Analysis: Per Serving
Calories 184, Fiber 5 gm, Cholesterol 0 mg, Sodium 328 mg, Percent of calories from: Protein 9%, Carbohydrate 68%, Fat 23% (5 gm fat)

Smoked Fish Pasta Salad

3 oz smoked salmon or trout, sliced thin and cut into pieces

2 cups cooked pasta (twist ties if available), drained

1 cup asparagus tips, cooked (canned are fine, if available)

1 cup raw, sliced summer squash

1/4 cup green onions, chopped

1/2 avocado, sliced (optional)

1 tsp dill

Pepper to taste

1/4 cup of your favorite reduced-calorie creamy bottled dressing

Mix all ingredients together gently. Makes 2 entree salad servings or 4 side salads.

Nutritional Analysis: Per Entree Salad

Calories 292, Fiber 4 gm, Cholesterol 30 mg, Sodium 840 mg, Percent of calories from: Protein 25%, Carbohydrate 59%, Fat 16%

Tabbouleh Salad

1/3 cup chopped walnuts or almonds

1 cup dry bulgur

2/3 cup chopped green onions

1 cup diced tomato (or quartered cherry tomatoes)

1/3 cup lemon juice

2 cups shredded romaine lettuce leaves

1/4 cup low-sodium chicken broth

Pepper to taste

Pour enough boiling water over bulgur to just cover. Let sit 30 minutes (until water is absorbed). Add remaining ingredients, except lettuce. Toss thoroughly. Cover and chill at least 2 hours. Toss in lettuce and serve. Makes 6 servings.

Nutritional Analysis: Per Serving

Calories 162, Fiber 4 gm, Cholesterol 0 mg, Sodium 40 mg, Percent of calories from: Protein 12%, Carbohydrate 63%, Fat 25%

Cucumber & Tomato Salad in Garlic Yogurt Dressing

1 lb cucumbers (about 2 medium), peeled and sliced

1/2 lb tomatoes, chopped

4 scallions, minced

1/2 cup fresh mint, chopped fine

1/2 cup fresh parsley, chopped fine

3 Tbsp lemon juice

2 cloves garlic, crushed

1 cup plain low-fat yogurt

Black pepper to taste

Mix the lemon juice, yogurt, garlic, pepper, mint, and parsley together. Pour over cucumber and tomato mixture and stir. Serve within one hour for best taste. Makes 6 servings.

Nutritional Analysis: Per Serving

Calories 45, Fiber 1 gm, Cholesterol 2 mg, Sodium 35 mg, Percent of calories from: Protein 24%, Carbohydrate 63%, Fat 13%

Chicken Salad Tropicale

5 cups cooked rice

4 leftover BBQ chicken breasts, boneless, skinless, and shredded into bite-sized pieces

1 (8-oz.) can unsweetened crushed pineapple, drained, but reserve the juice

2 cups jicama, finely chopped, or use sliced water chestnuts

2/3 cup green onions, finely chopped

2 1/2 cups celery, sliced

1/2 cup roasted peanuts (or other nuts)

spinach or romaine lettuce

Tropical Dressing:

1 cup plain low-fat yogurt

1 cup reduced-calories mayonnaise

2 to 3 Tbsp pineapple juice

1/4 cup honey

2 tsp finely grated fresh ginger

In large bowl, combine rice, chicken, pineapple, jicama, onions, and celery. In another bowl, blend all dressing ingredients until smooth. Pour dressing over rice mixture and toss. Serve on a bed of spinach or romaine lettuce leaves and sprinkle with roasted peanuts. Serves at least 12. This can be made a day in advance.

Nutritional Analysis: Per Serving
Calories 275, Fiber 2 gm, Cholesterol 30 mg, Sodium 160 mg, Percent of calories from: Protein 20%, Carbohydrate 53%, Fat 27%

❖ Side Dishes ❖

Seasoned Rice

1 cup uncooked brown rice

1 1/2 cup water

1 packet low-sodium chicken bouillon (or 1 cube)

1 cup chopped onion

1 1/2 cups vegetable pieces (grated carrots, broccoli, or a
combination of others)

2 tsp parsley flakes

1/2 lemon, sliced (used as garnish when serving, great
squeezed on top of the rice)

Mix low-sodium chicken bouillon with water in a medium saucepan. Add
the rice, onions, parsley, and mix. Spoon the vegetable pieces on top and
cover saucepan. Bring to a boil. Then reduce heat to a simmer. Let simmer
until rice is cooked and most of the water is gone (about 25 minutes). Stir
vegetables into the rest of the rice mixture and serve. Serves 4.

Nutritional Analysis: Per Serving
Calories 195, Fiber 6 gm, Cholesterol 0 mg, Sodium 25 mg, Percent of
calories from: Protein 10%, Carbohydrate 845, Fat 6%

Au Gratin Potatoes-Revised

4 potatoes, sliced into 1/8" thick slices

1 1/2 cup thinly sliced sweet or mild onion

1/2 cup low sodium chicken broth or beer

5 ounces reduced fat sharp cheddar cheese, grated

3 Tbsp flour

1 1/2 cup 1% low-fat milk

1 Tbsp parsley flakes

1 1/2 tsp oregano

Pepper to taste

Salt to taste

Topping:

3 Tbsp grated Parmesan or Romano cheese

1/4 cup cornflake crumbs

1 Tbsp diet margarine, melted

Preheat oven to 350°. Simmer onion rings in chicken broth or beer until nicely brown and tender. Drain and set aside. Layer half of the potato slices in 9 x 9" baking dish and top with half of onions. Sprinkle half of grated cheese over the top. Sprinkle half of the flour and seasonings over the top. Repeat with remainder of potatoes, onions, cheese, flour, and seasonings. Pour milk evenly over the top. Combine topping ingredients in small bowl and sprinkle evenly over the top. Cover loosely with foil and for 25 to 30 minutes until potatoes are cooked throughout. Makes 6 large side dish servings.

Nutritional Analysis: Per Serving (original recipe values)

Calories 309 (442), Fiber 4 gm, Cholesterol 18 mg (33 mg), Sodium 295 mg (will vary by taste), Percent of calories from: Protein 18% (11%), Carbohydrate 61% (45%), Fat 21% (43%), (7 gm of fat compared with 21.5 gm)

Oil-Free Hash Browns

2 cups red potatoes, chopped in 1/3-inch cubes, or buy frozen Southern
  style hash browns
1 1/2 cups water
1 packet (or cube) low-sodium chicken bouillon
1/2 cup chopped onion
1 or 2 cloves garlic
1 Tbsp parsley flakes

Optional: 1/3 cup grated sharp cheddar cheese

Heat water and bouillon powder, onion, garlic, parsley, and potatoes in
medium saucepan until boiling. Drop to medium heat and let simmer,
uncovered, until water evaporates and potatoes are tender (about 15 minutes). Add cheese if desired. Makes 2 servings.

Nutritional Analysis: Per Serving (with cheese)
Calories 255, Fiber 6 gm, Cholesterol 20 mg, Sodium 220 mg, Percent of
calories from: Protein 16%, Carbohydrate 62%, Fat 22%

Country Bread Stuffing

12 ounces turkey breakfast sausage (or other ground meat)

2 cups onions, chopped

2 cups mushrooms, sliced

2 cups celery, chopped

1 stick butter or margarine (1/2 cup)

2 cups grated carrots

4 cups low-sodium chicken broth

21 ounces Pepperidge Farms® Herb-Seasoned Stuffing (or similar bread cubes with almost no fat added)

2 Tbsp parsley flakes

Heat sausage for about 4 minutes on medium heat in large Teflon frying pan, breaking up meat into pieces. Add onions, celery, mushrooms, and butter. After sausage browns and vegetables become tender, add grated carrots and parsley. Heat for another couple of minutes, stirring frequently.

While you are waiting for the sausage-vegetable mixture to cook, boil 4 cups of chicken broth in a large saucepan. Remove pan from heat and pour in 21 ounces of stuffing cubes, stirring quickly to evenly moisten the stuffing with broth. When vegetable-sausage mixture is cooked throughout, add to bread cubes and stir well.

To finish cooking or to reheat later, place saucepan on low heat for about 20 minutes, stirring often. Makes about 12 servings.

Nutritional Analysis: Per Serving

Calories 295, Fiber 1.5 gm, Cholesterol 35 mg, Sodium up to 1000 mg (depending on bread cubes), Percent of calories from: Protein 18%, Carbohydrate 48%, Fat 34%

Carrots with Apricots

1 cup dried apricots

3 cups carrots, cut into 1/2" rounds

3 Tbsp water

1 tsp butter or margarine

Pinch of sugar

Chopped fresh parsley or dill for garnish

Soak apricots in hot water for 1 1/2 hours to soften or microwave in water on high for a minute or two. Pat dry and cut in julienne strips. In a skillet or frying pan with a tightly fitting lid, combine carrots, water, margarine, and sugar. Cover and cook over medium heat for 12 to 15 minutes or until carrots are tender. Stir occasionally to prevent sticking. Stir in apricots and heat through. Serve garnished with parsley or dill. Serves 4.

Nutritional Analysis: Per Serving

Calories 70, Fiber 1 gm, Cholesterol 0, Sodium 46 mg, Percent of calories from: Protein 7%, Carbohydrate 85%, Fat 8%

Broccoli Rice Parmesan

2 cups broccoli florets, chopped raw

1 cup uncooked rice (brown or white)

2 cups 1% low-fat milk

1/4 cup chopped green onions

1/4 cup grated Parmesan cheese

1 Tbsp diet margarine

2 packets low-sodium chicken or beef broth powder (Herb-Ox)

In medium saucepan, add 1 1/2 cup milk and 1/2 cup water, rice, broth powder, and margarine. Cover and bring to boil, then reduce to simmer. While waiting for the rice and milk to boil, chop green onions and broccoli florets into small, bite-sized pieces. Once you reduce the rice-milk mixture to a simmer, add the broccoli and onions on top. Cover and simmer about 20 more minutes until rice is done. Mix in 1/2 cup remaining milk and Parmesan. Makes 4 servings.

Nutritional Analysis: Per Serving
Calories 180, Fiber 2 gm (with white rice), Cholesterol 10 mg, Sodium 230 mg, Percent of calories from: Protein 17%, Carbohydrate 65%, Fat 18% (5.5 gm fat)

Elaine's French Fries

2 large russet potatoes (or 3 medium)

1 tsp vegetable oil

Salt as desired (analyzed without salt)

Seasoning suggestions: garlic, finely chopped or Italian herbs, or if you like it hot, try some chili powder, cayenne red pepper, or paprika.

Preheat oven to 400°. Cut potatoes into shoestring-sized strips. Using a plastic spatula, spread the oil evenly on Teflon baking sheet. Lay potatoes in a single layer on sheet. Bake for 10 to 15 minutes or until lightly brown. Flip potatoes to other side with spatula, sprinkle salt or other seasonings on top if desired, and bake about 10 minutes more. Makes 2 large servings.

Nutritional Analysis: Per Serving (without added salt)

Calories 160, Fiber 4 gm, Cholesterol 0 mg, Sodium 2 mg, Percent of calories from: Protein 9%, Carbohydrate 78%, Fat 13%

❖ Sandwiches ❖

Chicken Sandwich with Salsa

1 chicken breast, cooked, without skin

1 French roll

Green leaf lettuce

About 1/8 cup salsa

Nutritional Analysis: Per Sandwich

Calories 450, Cholesterol 70 mg, Sodium up to 700 mg, depending on salsa, Percent of calories from fat, 12%

Special Turkey Sandwich

3 ounces cooked turkey breast (use smoked, if desired)

1/8 cup cranberry sauce

Green leaf lettuce

1 French roll

Nutritional Analysis: Per Sandwich

Calories 450, Cholesterol 60 mg, Sodium 580 mg, Percent of calories from: Protein 30%, Carbohydrate 57%, Fat 13%

Lowered Cholesterol
Egg Salad Sandwich

6 large eggs

2 Tbsp reduced-calorie mayonnaise

1/4 cup chopped green onions

1/4 cup finely chopped celery

Pepper to taste

Dijon mustard, to taste (optional)

1 tomato, sliced

dark green lettuce leaves

8 slices whole-wheat bread

Set eggs in medium saucepan, cover with water. Heat to a boil. Let boil for 5 minutes. Let eggs cool, then remove shells. Remove 3 of the yolks and throw them away. Take a fork and gently shred the remaining whole eggs and 3 egg whites. Stir in the reduced-calorie mayonnaise, onion, and celery. Then add pepper and mustard to taste. Spread on slices of bread and garnish with tomato and lettuce. Makes 4 sandwiches.

Nutritional Analysis: Per Sandwich

Calories 265, Fiber 5 gm, Cholesterol about 150 mg, Sodium, 480 mg, Percent of calories from: Protein 19%, Carbohydrate 58%, Fat 23%

Lite Chicken Salad Sandwich

4 boneless, skinless chicken breasts, cut into bite-sized chunks

2 cups low-sodium chicken broth

1/2 cup diced jicama (or water chestnuts)

1 green onion, finely chopped

1/4 cup and 1 Tbsp plain low-fat yogurt

1 1/2 tsp Dijon mustard

1 tsp parsley flakes

1/2 tsp dill

pepper to taste

1/4 cup grated sharp cheddar cheese

2 whole tomatoes, sliced

1/2 whole cucumber, sliced

12 slices sourdough bread (or whole-wheat)

Sauté chicken chunks in 2 cups chicken broth until thoroughly cooked. Drain and let cool. Mix yogurt, mustard, onion, parsley, and dill together well. Add chicken chunks, cheese, and pepper to taste. Serve on bread with slices of tomato and cucumber. Makes 6 sandwiches.

Nutritional Analysis: Per Sandwich

Calories 250, Fiber 1 gm, Cholesterol 6 mg, Sodium 620 mg, Percent of calories from: Protein 15%, Carbohydrate 70%, Fat 15%

❖ Breakfast Entrees ❖

Buttermilk-Oatmeal Pancakes

1 1/4 cup buttermilk

1 Tbsp oil

1 egg, beaten with 2 egg whites

1 Tbsp honey

1 cup rolled oats

1/2 cup whole-wheat flour

1/2 tsp baking soda

1/2 tsp cinnamon

Combine the buttermilk and rolled oats in a bowl and let stand about 5 minutes. In another bowl, stir the dry ingredients together. Add eggs, oil, and honey to the bowl with buttermilk and oats. Add dry ingredients to wet. Stir to moisten. Pour 1/4 cup batter for each pancake into medium hot Teflon pan. Turn pancakes when top is bubbly and edges are slightly dry. (Be patient, these pancakes take a bit longer to cook because of the oats.) Makes 3 large servings.

Topping Ideas: Try to skip the butter and add instead: pureed fruits, non- or low-sugar preserves, light syrups, or plain yogurt with chopped apples and almonds or bananas and pecans.

Nutritional Analysis: Per Serving
Calories 310, Fiber 4 gm, Cholesterol 90 mg, Sodium 300 mg, Percent of calories from: Protein 15%, Carbohydrate 55%, Fat 26%

Low-Fat Pigs in Blankets

4 ounces cooked turkey breakfast sausage links
   (about 5 1/2 oz uncooked)

1/4 cup Aunt Jemima Buckwheat Pancake and Waffle Mix
   (or similar "incomplete" whole-grain mix)

1/4 cup Aunt Jemima Buttermilk Pancake and Waffle mix
   (or similar "incomplete" mix)

1/2 cup nonfat milk

1 egg white

Separate the raw turkey sausage into 6 links and cook over medium heat in a large frying pan. While meat is cooking, mix the pancake mixes together, add egg white and milk, and beat well. (Do not follow the directions on the box.) When sausage is cooked throughout and edges are browned, set aside. Make 3 pancakes, using 1/2 the batter. Repeat with remaining batter. Serve 3 pancakes with 3 links to make a serving, wrapping each link in a pancake. This recipe makes 2 servings. Serve with fresh fruit or juice to bring down the percentage of calories from fat.

Nutritional Analysis: Per Serving

Calories 265, Fiber and cholesterol information not available on product labels, Sodium 1090 mg, Percent of calories from: Protein 29%, Carbohydrate 41%, Fat 30%

❖ Lunch and Dinner Entrees ❖

Italian Style Hamburgers or Meatballs

12 to 14 ounces of ground sirloin (less than 13% fat)
4 green onions, chopped
1 egg white
1/4 tsp black pepper
3 cloves garlic, minced (optional)
1/3 cup fresh parsley, finely chopped
5 Tbsp cracker meal or Italian Seasoned bread crumbs

For Hamburgers: Mix ingredients well with a large spoon. Pat into 4 burgers. Grill or fry (not adding any extra fat) until cooked throughout. Serve on a bun or with slices of bread. Add dark green lettuce leaves and tomato for freshness. Moisten bread with a bit of catsup or mustard if you like.

Nutritional Analysis: Per Hamburger with Bun
Calories 355, Cholesterol 60 mg, Sodium 340 mg, Percent of calories from: Protein 29%, Carbohydrate 43%, Fat 28%

For Meatballs: Mix ingredients together well with large spoon. Roll by hand into about 50 meatballs. Over medium heat, cook in large frying pan until brown on all sides and cooked throughout. Serve as an hors d'oeuvre or toss into a tomato sauce and serve with pasta. Makes 50 meatballs (about 10 servings).

Nutritional Analysis: Per 5 Meatballs
Calories 90, Fiber 1 gm, Cholesterol 25 mg, Sodium 50 mg, Percent of calories from: Protein 41%, Carbohydrate 26%, Fat 33%

Sausage-Potato Shepherd's Pie

5 medium potatoes (or 3 large)

1 packet Butter Buds powder (1/2 oz)

3 Tbsp Parmesan cheese (optional)

3 Tbsp 1% (low-fat) milk

6 to 8 oz turkey breakfast sausage

1/2 cup carrot coins

1 cup corn

1/4 tsp celery seed

1/2 tsp basil leaves

1 tsp parsley flakes

pepper to taste

2 oz part-skim cheese, grated

Preheat oven to 400°. Cook potatoes in microwave until tender, then mash with milk, butter buds, and Parmesan cheese (peel potatoes first, if desired). Cook sausage until nicely browned; break into small pieces. Microwave carrots and corn until almost tender (about 2 to 3 minutes). Pat half of potato mixture into a lightly greased one-quart casserole dish. In medium-sized bowl, mix together sausage, carrots, and corn, and herbs. Spoon evenly into potato crust-lined dish. Cover with grated cheese. Pat remaining potato mixture evenly over the top. Bake for 30 minutes. Makes 4 entree servings.

Nutritional Analysis: Per Serving
Calories 390, Fiber 5 gm, Cholesterol (not available), Percent of calories from: Protein 17%, Carbohydrate 56%, Fat 27%

Fish Sticks

13 oz. Sea Bass, raw (or other thick and firm white fish)
1/2 cup cracker meal or crumbs
1/4 tsp pepper
1/2 tsp Italian seasonings
1 tsp parsley flakes
2 egg whites mixed with 3 Tbsp low-fat milk
2 tsp oil

Preheat oven to 375°. Cut fish into 1/2-inch thick sticks (about 2 to 3 inches in length and about an inch in width). In a medium-sized bowl, mix cracker meal with spices. Beat egg white with milk in another medium-sized bowl and set aside. Coat a Teflon baking sheet with the oil. With fork, dip and coat each fish piece in the egg-white mixture, then in the crumb mixture. Place them on baking sheet. Bake until golden brown—about 15 minutes. (You may need to flip them over to brown the other side.) Serve with spicy mustard or catsup. (Stay away from the fatty tartar sauces and mayonnaise.) Makes 3 servings.

Nutritional Analysis: Per Serving
Calories 245, Fiber 0.6 gm, Cholesterol 63 mg, Sodium 110 mg, Percent of calories from: Protein 48%, Carbohydrate 28%, Fat 24%

Broiled Fish with Tomato

3 Orange Roughy fillets (12 ounces, raw)
  or other boneless white fish, such as sole or snapper
1 tomato, sliced

Broiling Sauce:

2 Tbsp Oriental Chef-Delicate Sesame salad dressing or similar bottled
  salad dressing
1 tsp reduced-sodium soy sauce
1 tsp honey

Lay fish fillets on foil-covered baking sheet. Gently spoon half of broiling
sauce evenly over fish. Broil for several minutes, watching carefully. Flip
fillets over. Place tomato slices around fish fillets and dress both with the
remaining sauce. Continue broiling until fish is cooked throughout. Makes
3 servings.

Nutritional Analysis: Per Serving
Calories 135, Sodium 280 mg, Percent of calories from: Protein 62%,
Carbohydrate 16%, Fat 22%

Salmon with
Sour Cream Dill Sauce

2 salmon fillets or steaks (14 to 16 ounces)

1 cup White Zinfandel wine (or similar)

1 1/2 tsp cornstarch

2 Tbsp light sour cream

1 1/2 tsp lemon juice

1/8 tsp dill weed

Poach salmon fillets in a large covered saucepan by adding 1 cup Zinfandel wine and simmering over medium heat until just cooked throughout (about 10 minutes) or until fish flakes with a fork. Lift fish from pan and place on a serving platter or dinner plates. Reduce heat to a simmer. In a small cup, mix cornstarch with the sour cream. Stir mixture into remaining Zinfandel in saucepan. Add in lemon juice and dill weed. Stir until smooth and thickened. Drizzle over salmon fillets. Makes 2 large servings.

Nutritional Analysis: Per Serving

Calories 410, Cholesterol 120 mg, Sodium 112 mg, Percent of calories from: Protein 44%, Carbohydrate 4%, Fat 32% (14.5 gm fat)

Seafood with Lemon Sauce

2 tsp margarine

2 Tbsp lemon juice

1 clove garlic

1 tsp basil flakes, crushed in hand while added

4 Tbsp champagne or white wine

2 tsp cornstarch

1 Tbsp low-fat milk

16 oz raw scallops

Pepper to taste

4 cups cooked pasta

Melt margarine with garlic over medium-high heat. Brown for about a minute. Add scallops, lemon juice, champagne, basil, and pepper. Cover and let cook for a few minutes.

Meanwhile, mix milk and cornstarch. When scallops are almost tender throughout, add milk mixture, stir, then lower heat to a simmer. Let cook, uncovered, for a couple minutes more. Serve over pasta. Makes 4 servings.

Nutritional Analysis: Per Serving
Calories 300, Cholesterol 43 mg, Sodium 320 mg, Percent of calories from: Protein 33%, Carbohydrate 57%, Fat 10%

Beef Tacos

8 corn tortillas

7 oz uncooked lean ground beef
  (Use ground sirloin with less than 13% fat, if available.)

1/2 cup onions, chopped

1 cup canned kidney beans, drained

1/4 to 1/2 tsp chili con carne seasoning

pepper to taste (1/4 to 1/2 tsp)

1 grated carrot

2 tomatoes, diced

1 cup grated part-skim cheese (use less to lower fat)

2 cups leaf lettuce, shredded

Add beef, onions, and seasonings to Teflon fry pan and cook over medium heat until meat is done throughout. Add beans and let simmer a couple minutes longer. Soften tortillas by placing each one in a Teflon fry pan over medium heat. Flip to other side and continue heating. Then remove and repeat with other tortillas. Fill tortillas with beef, carrot, tomatoes, cheese, and lettuce. Makes 4 servings (2 tacos each).

Nutritional Analysis: Per Serving
Calories 390, Fiber 11 gm, Cholesterol 40 mg, Sodium 225 mg, Percent of calories from: Protein 25%, Carbohydrate 45%, Fat 30%

Enchilada Pie

1 lb lean ground beef (ground sirloin, Healthy Choice®
   ground beef)

1 1/2 cup canned or cooked kidney or pinto beans

6 corn tortillas

1 small clove garlic (minced) or 1/8 tsp garlic powder

1/2 medium onion (chopped)

1/4 tsp chili powder

1 small can (3 oz.) diced green chilies

1/2 can Campbell's Healthy Request Cream of Mushroom Soup,
   condensed

1 can (14.5 oz.) S & W Mexican Style Stewed Tomatoes

6 ounces reduced fat sharp cheddar cheese (Cracker Barrel or Kraft
   Light N' Natural), grated

Crumble ground beef into heated skillet. Add garlic, onion, and chili powder. Cook over moderate heat, stirring occasionally. Add beans, drained of
any liquid, and stir. Mix 1/2 a can of condensed mushroom soup (do not
add water) with a can of stewed tomatoes. Layer half of meat/bean mixture
in the bottom of an 8 x 8 nonstick baking pan (or similar). Top with half of
tomato mixture. Layer half of corn tortillas evenly over the top. (Cut them
in half to make them fit if need be). Sprinkle grated cheese over the top.
Repeat with layers of meat, sauce, tortillas, and cheese. Cover loosely with
foil and bake in 350° oven for 45 minutes. Makes 6 servings.

Nutritional Analysis: per serving
Calories 347, Fiber 4 gm, Cholesterol 59 mg, Sodium 684 mg, Percent of
calories from: Protein 34%, Carbohydrate 37%, Fat 29% (11 gm fat)

Last-Minute Chili

1 tsp oil

2 Tbsp whiskey or Brandy

9 to 10 ounces braised beef tips (small cubes)

2 large garlic cloves, minced

1 yellow onion, coarsely chopped

2 cups eggplant, cut into small cubes

2 tsp dried parsley flakes (crumble while adding)

1 tsp. dried oregano

1 tsp chili con carne seasoning

Black pepper, to taste (about 1/2 tsp)

2 (14.5 oz each) cans stewed Mexican style tomatoes

2 (15.5 oz each) cans kidney beans, drained and rinsed well

2 Tbsp tomato paste

In a large nonstick skillet, heat oil and garlic over medium-high heat. Add beef cubes and let fry for a minute, stirring constantly. Add whiskey and stir. Then add onions and eggplant. Let simmer a minute. Add spices and lower heat to medium low. Add the tomatoes and juice, tomato paste, and beans. Cover and let simmer 30 minutes. Stir occasionally. Makes 6 servings.

Nutritional Analysis: Per Serving

Calories 270, Fiber 14 gm, Cholesterol 32 mg, Sodium 720 mg (would be much lower if low-salt tomatoes and beans are used), Percent of calories from: Protein 32%, Carbohydrate 55%, Fat 14% (4 gm)

Generic Stir Fry

2 tsp sesame oil

2 to 3 Tbsp low-sodium chicken broth or white wine

2 chicken breasts, skinned and boned, cut into cubes (or use 7 oz shell-fish, turkey, or lean beef cuts)

1 clove garlic, minced

1 or 2 slices fresh ginger, chopped (or 1/8 tsp powdered)

1/2 cup low-sodium chicken broth

3 cups vegetables (your choice)

1 1/2 tsp reduced-sodium soy sauce

1 to 2 tsp cornstarch, dissolved in a little water

3 cups cooked brown rice

Heat wok or large Teflon frying pan until very hot. Add oil, turning pan to coat. Add chicken pieces, 2 to 3 tablespoons chicken broth, garlic, and gin-ger, stirring constantly until chicken is white. Add more broth if more mois-ture is needed. Remove chicken and set aside.

Add the rest of the chicken broth and any "long cooking" vegetables, such as carrots, broccoli, or cauliflower. Bring to a boil. Cook about 4 minutes, stir-ring constantly. Add any medium-cooking vegetables, such as green peppers or squash, and cooked chicken. Stir and cook about 2 minutes. Add any quick-cooking vegetables (bok choy, spinach leaves, bean sprouts) and soy sauce. Stir vegetables for a minute or two. Add more chicken broth if more moisture is needed. Thicken by pushing the vegetables to one side and stir-ring in the cornstarch mixture. Heat and stir until thickened. Stir in the veg-etables to coat with sauce. Serve on bed of cooked rice. Makes 3 servings.

Nutritional Analysis: Per Serving: (Analyzed with 1 1/2 cup broccoli and 1 1/2 cups carrots)
Calories 395, Fiber 13 gm, Cholesterol 47 mg, Sodium 290 mg, Percent of calories from: Protein 26%, Carbohydrate 58%, Fat 16%

Lemon Chicken Parmesan

1 1/2 oz dried tomato slices (add warm water and set aside for 20 minutes to reconstitute slightly)

4 skinless, boneless chicken breasts

1 lemon

1/2 tsp black pepper

1 tsp dried rosemary flakes or 2 tsp dried basil leaves
(crush in hand while adding)

Cheese Sauce:

1 cup part-skim ricotta cheese

1/2 cup nonfat milk

2/3 cup Parmesan cheese

Serve over 6 cups cooked pasta (about 9 oz fresh pasta)

Place dried tomato slices in 9-inch square baking dish to make a bed for the chicken breasts. Add chicken breasts evenly, laying completely flat. Squeeze juice of 1 lemon over all of the chicken. Sprinkle pepper and basil or rosemary on top. Cover dish with foil and bake in preheated 350° oven until tender (about 45 minutes). Mix cheese sauce in microwave-safe dish. Microwave on high for 2 minutes until hot and bubbly. Pour over chicken when done. Bake uncovered for 5 minutes. Broil for the last minute or so to lightly brown the top, if desired. Serve each portion over 1 1/2 cups cooked pasta. Makes 4 servings.

Nutritional Analysis: Per Serving
Calories 590, Fiber 3 gm, Cholesterol 100 mg, Sodium 455 mg, Percent of calories from: Protein 34%, Carbohydrate 45%, Fat 21%

Dijon Chicken

About 1 lb raw boneless, skinless, chicken breasts

1 Tbsp butter or margarine

3/4 cup white wine

2 leeks, white part only, thinly sliced

3 Tbsp Dijon-style mustard

2 Tbsp evaporated low-fat milk mixed with 1 Tbsp flour

3 cups cooked brown rice (or white, if you prefer)

Cut chicken breasts into 1/2-inch strips. Sauté in 1 tablespoon butter and 1/2 cup wine until cooked throughout (about 4 to 5 minutes). Remove chicken pieces with a slotted spoon. Sauté leeks in pan drippings for about 3 minutes. Add the rest of the wine, mustard, milk, and flour mixture and simmer until the sauce thickens slightly (about 5 minutes), stirring frequently. Add chicken chunks. Serve over rice. Makes 3 servings.

Nutritional Analysis: Per Serving
Calories 530, Fiber 5 gm, Cholesterol 105 mg, Sodium 343 mg, Percent of calories from: Protein 35%, Carbohydrate 45%, Fat 20%

Quick Quesadillas

2 flour tortillas

1/2 cup grated part-skim cheese of choice

1 Tbsp tomato sauce, salsa, or bottled spaghetti sauce

1/4 cup chopped green onions

1/2 cup chopped fresh tomatoes

1/4 cup low-fat plain yogurt

In a Teflon pan, heat both sides of one tortilla until it is soft and hot. Spread 2 tablespoons of sauce down the middle of the tortilla. Sprinkle half the grated cheese evenly over the tortilla, followed with onions and tomatoes. When tortilla browns and cheese starts to bubble, fold one side toward the middle and then fold the other side. Top with 1/8 cup yogurt. Repeat with rest of ingredients.

Nutritional Analysis: Per Quesadilla

Calories 215, Fiber 1.5 gm, Cholesterol 45 mg, Sodium 480 mg, Percent of calories from: Protein 24%, Carbohydrate 43%, Fat 33%

Lard-Less, Low-Fat
Chicken Tamales

1 pkg dried corn husks

1/2 cup diet margarine

1/2 cup nonfat ricotta cheese

1/3 cup nonfat sour cream

2 packets low sodium chicken or beef bouillon

4 cups Masa Harina corn tortilla flour

1 tsp salt

2 2/3 cups low sodium chicken or beef broth (or water)

Chicken or beef filling (for a quick chicken filling, see recipe below)

For Masa: With hand mixer, whip margarine, ricotta cheese, sour cream, and low-sodium chicken bouillon powder in medium-sized bowl until fluffy. By hand, or on the lowest speed of the electric mixer, blend in 4 cups Masa flour, 1 teaspoon salt, and 2 2/3 cups warm broth. Mix until dough holds together well. Use dough immediately or refrigerate up to 3 days (bring to room temperature before using).

For Husks: In large roasting pan, cover husks with warm water and let stand until pliable (about 30 minutes). Drain and pat dry when ready to use. For each tamale, select a wide, pliable husk. Lay flat, with tip pointing away from you. Form a rectangle by spreading two level tablespoons of masa down the center of husk (3 inches from the tip and 1 inch from one side and bottom of husk). Spoon two rounded tablespoons of filling in center of Masa. Envelope filling by folding husk so Masa edges meet. The plain edge wraps around the outside of the tamale. Fold the bottom end of the husk up around the tamale and fold down the tip. Set each tamale, seam side down, in a holding container, or set on a tray and cover with a damp cloth. Continue until all filling and masa is used.

To Steam: Fill 12- to 14-quart pan or steamer with an inch of boiling water. Put in steamer rack (a metal vegetable steamer can be used). Stack tamales in steamer with some space in between so heat can circulate. Bring water to a boil, then cover and lower heat to maintain a steady boil. Continue steaming for about one hour, adding boiling water to keep the water level at one inch. When done, masa should be firm and the husk easy to peel away. Makes at least 30 tamales.

Quick Chicken Filling

4 chicken breasts, skinless

4 to 5 chicken thighs, skinless

1 1/2 cups chopped onion

1/2 cup nonalcoholic beer (or something similar)

2 to 3 cups low-sodium chicken broth

1 1/4 cups canned enchilada sauce

2 Tbsp chopped black olives

1 pickled jalapeno or other small chili, stemmed and finely minced (optional)

On low boil, cook chicken in chicken broth. When cooked throughout, shred by hand into bite-sized pieces (remove any remaining bone or skin). Heat 1/2 cup nonalcoholic beer or wine in frying pan. Add onion and cook until soft (about 5 minutes). Stir in chicken pieces, olives, enchilada sauce, and minced chili. Reduce heat to simmer and cook, uncovered, for 10 minutes, stirring occasionally.

Nutritional Analysis: Per Tamale
Calories 128, Fiber 2.5 gm, Cholesterol 16 mg, Sodium 30 mg, Percent of calories from: Protein 26%, Carbohydrate 46%, Fat 28% (4 gm of fat)

Ground Beef Tostadas

4 flour or large corn tortillas (9" dia.), baked or pan fried until crisp

4 oz. shredded reduced fat Jack or Cheddar cheese

4 cups shredded lettuce

2 medium tomatoes, chopped or sliced

Optional garnishes: nonfat or light sour cream, green onions, salsa, beans, or, but go light on: avocados, extra cheese, olives

For beef filling:

1 lb. ground sirloin or Healthy Choice® beef

1 medium onion, chopped

2 cloves garlic, minced or pressed

1 1/2 tsp chili powder

1 tsp paprika

1 tsp oregano

1/4 tsp ground cumin

Pepper to taste (about 1/4 tsp)

1/2 cup canned tomato sauce or mild chili sauce

2 tsp Worcestershire sauce

Over medium-high heat, crumble beef in large nonstick frying pan. Add onion and garlic and cook, stirring frequently, until meat is browned and cooked throughout. Stir in remaining filling ingredients and simmer on low until thickened.

To assemble: Place tortillas on plates and top with layers of meat, cheese, lettuce, tomato, and optional garnishes. Makes 4 servings.

Nutritional Analysis: Per Serving
Calories 395, Fiber 6 gm, Cholesterol 91 mg, Sodium 406 mg, Percent of calories from: Protein 39%, Carbohydrate 31%, Fat 30% (13 gm fat)

At-Home Fajitas

4 fajita flour tortillas

12 oz raw chicken breast, round steak, skirt steak, or swordfish

Marinade:

1 cup low-sodium chicken broth

1 Tbsp soy sauce

1 tsp Worcestershire sauce

1 clove garlic, finely chopped

1/2 tsp pepper

1 tsp lemon juice

Salsa Guacamole:

1/2 avocado, mashed

3 Tbsp plain low-fat yogurt (or nonfat)

2 cups leaf lettuce, shredded

1 cup chopped tomatoes

Cut meat in 1/3-inch-thick strips. Mix marinade and add meat to it. Marinate for about 4 hours in the refrigerator. (If you're out of time, skip the marinate time.) Make guacamole mixture and set aside in a serving bowl. Remove meat strips and set in Teflon fry pan with half the marinade. (Throw the other half away.) Simmer until the meat is well done and the marinade has almost boiled off. Quickly remove meat into a serving bowl. To soften tortillas, place in nonstick fry pan on medium-high heat and flip to other side when lightly brown and soft. Makes 4 fajitas.

Nutritional Analysis: Per Chicken Fajita (Round Steak values are in parentheses)

Calories 260 (275), Fiber 2 gm, Cholesterol 53 mg (56 mg), Sodium 470 mg (this will be much less if reduced-sodium soy sauce is used), Percent of calories from: Protein 37% (35%), Carbohydrate 35% (33%), Fat 28% (32%)

Tuna Enchiladas

4 corn tortillas

1 (6.5 oz) can solid white tuna, water packed, drained

2 Tbsp green onion, chopped

1/2 cup grated part-skim cheese

1/3 cup Ragu Gardenstyle spaghetti sauce

1/8 tsp chili powder

1 (more) cup Ragu Gardenstyle spaghetti sauce

1/2 cup plain low-fat yogurt

6 black olives, cut in half

Preheat oven to 375°. Mix tuna with green onions, cheese, 1/3 cup sauce, and chili powder. Heat each tortilla in a Teflon pan to soften. Spread remaining cup of spaghetti sauce in baking pan. Roll 1/4 of tuna mixture in one tortilla and repeat with remaining 3 tortillas. Place in pan. Bake for 10 to 15 minutes. Cool a couple of minutes before serving. Top each enchilada with 2 Tbsp yogurt and 3 olive halves. Serves 2.

Nutritional Analysis: Per Serving

Calories 473, Fiber 6 gm, Cholesterol 85 mg, Sodium 705 mg, Percent of calories from: Protein 36%, Carbohydrate 38%, Fat 26%

Quick and Light Chilies Rellenos

12 oz whole fire-roasted green chilies (eg., Ortega)

6 to 8 oz reduced fat Jack cheese, cut into 1/4-inch thick slices

1/2 cup flour

2 Tbsp low-chicken broth or beer

1 small onion, chopped

1 to 2 cloves garlic, minced or pressed

1 1/2 cups no-salt tomato puree

1/2 tsp oregano

Crispy egg coating:

4 egg whites, 2 yolks, 1/4 cup egg substitute, 1/2 tsp salt

about 1 Tbsp oil for pan frying

Drain chilies and select the biggest and best ones. Insert each chili with a slice or two of cheese. Roll chilies generously in flour and set aside. In medium fry pan, add broth, onion, and garlic, cooking and stirring until lightly brown. Add tomato puree and oregano. Season with salt or pepper, if desired. Reduce heat, cover, and simmer for 10 minutes.

For crispy egg coating, in large bowl, whip egg whites with 1/2 teaspoon salt until firm peaks form. In separate bowl, beat yolks with egg substitute until blended. Fold quickly into whipped egg whites. Start heating nonstick fry pan. Pour in about 2 teaspoons oil. While oil is getting hot, dip cheese-filled chilies into egg coating and place in pan. Quickly repeat dipping until bottom of pan is filled with chilies. With spoon, spread a little of egg batter mixture on the top of chilies that have lost a little of their batter. After about 1 or 2 minutes, check bottoms; if golden, carefully turn over with a fork and spatula. When golden, remove chilies. Repeat procedure with remaining chilies. Serve immediately with sauce or bake rellenos with sauce and cheese garnish in baking dish just until warm. Makes 6 servings.

Nutritional Analysis: Per Serving
Calories 234, Fiber 4 gm, Cholesterol 89 mg, Sodium 1250 mg or less, Percent of calories from: Protein 27%, Carbohydrate 34%, Fat 39% (10 gm fat)

Chicken with Asparagus

4 chicken breasts, skinned and boned

1/2 cup cracker meal (cracker crumbs or flour)

1/4 tsp black pepper

1 tsp parsley flakes

1/2 tsp thyme

1/2 oz Butter Buds® (one small packet)

1 1/2 cups asparagus, cooked

2 1/2 cups pasta, cooked

Gravy:

1 1/2 cups low-sodium chicken broth

3/4 cup raw sliced mushrooms

1/3 cup diced onions

1 Tbsp margarine, melted

2 Tbsp flour

1/4 cup skim or low-fat milk

1/4 cup grated Parmesan cheese

Preheat oven to 400°. Mix cracker meal and seasonings together in a bowl. Mix up the Butter Buds, following directions on package, in a separate bowl. Dip chicken breasts in Butter Buds®, one at a time, then dip in crumb mixture and place on Teflon baking sheet. Bake for about 30 minutes, turning chicken after 15 minutes. While chicken is baking, boil pasta and asparagus and make gravy. Simmer mushrooms and onions in broth over medium-high heat until tender. Add margarine mixed with flour and cook until thickened. Add milk and simmer a few minutes longer until creamy.

When chicken is ready, arrange 4 nests of pasta on a serving dish and lay a chicken breast on each nest. Garnish the edges with cooked asparagus spears. Pour gravy evenly over chicken and pasta. Sprinkle top with Parmesan cheese. Serves 4.

Nutritional Analysis: Per Serving
Calories 395, Fiber 3 gm, Cholesterol 75 mg, Sodium 270 mg, Percent of calories from: Protein 37%, Carbohydrate 45%, Fat 18%

Chicken Pesto Wedding Lasagna

I made this lasagna for our wedding dinner.

4 boneless, skinless chicken breasts, cut into bite-sized pieces
1 packet low-sodium chicken broth mixed with 3/4 cup water
2 tsp Italian seasoning
2 cups grated zucchini
2/3 cup (5 oz) Pesto For Pasta (or other pesto), drained
1 1/2 cup part-skim ricotta cheese
1/2 cup Parmesan cheese
2/3 cup chopped green onions
12 oz (dry weight) lasagna noodles
8 oz part-skim mozzarella cheese, grated
2 1/2 cups Ragu Gardenstyle Spaghetti Sauce

Preheat oven to 375°. In frying pan, simmer chicken pieces in broth and Italian seasonings over medium heat until cooked. While chicken is cooking, mix the ricotta and Parmesan cheese with green onions in a bowl. Using a slotted spoon, remove chicken pieces from pan. Lightly shred chicken in food processor with pesto and zucchini. Cook noodles until just tender. To make lasagna, first spread 1 cup Ragu on bottom of 9 x 13-inch pan. Add 3 strips lasagna noodles. Spread on half the chicken mixture and add 3 strips lasagna on top. Then spread the cheese mixture and top with 3 strips lasagna. Then spread the rest of the chicken mixture and top with 3 strips lasagna. Spread 2 1/2 cups Ragu on top and sprinkle with the grated mozzarella. Bake for 25 minutes. Makes 12 servings.

Nutritional Analysis: Per Serving
Calories 335, Fiber (not available), Cholesterol 45 mg, Sodium 500 mg, Percent of calories from: Protein 28%, Carbohydrate 44%, Fat 28%

Slimmed-Down Fettucini Alfredo

1 Tbsp butter

1 small clove garlic, finely minced (Optional)

7/8 cup 1% low-fat milk (remove 2 Tbsp from 1 cup measure)

2 tsp flour for thickening

3 Tbsp grated Parmesan cheese

Pinch or two of nutmeg

3 cups cooked fettucini noodles

Heat butter and garlic in small nonstick fry pan over medium until garlic browns slightly. In small bowl, mix one tablespoon milk with the flour to make a paste. Stir in the rest of the milk and mix well. Add the milk mixture to browning butter and let bubble, stirring frequently, for a couple minutes. When sauce has thickened to your liking, turn off the heat and stir in the Parmesan cheese. Sprinkle the nutmeg (and freshly ground pepper if you like) evenly over the top. Spoon sauce over cooked, drained pasta. Makes 2 large servings.

Nutritional Analysis: Per Large Serving

Calories 395, Fiber 1 gm, Cholesterol 28 mg, Sodium 255 mg, Percent of calories from: Protein 16%, Carbohydrate 61%, Fat 23%

Spanakopita (Greek Spinach Pie)

9 sheets phyllo dough

1 1/2 Tbsp butter or margarine

8 ounces feta cheese

8 ounces nonfat ricotta cheese

1/2 bunch fresh green onions

1 medium onion

1/4 cup beer, wine, or broth

2 8-oz packages frozen spinach, chopped

1 egg and 1 egg white (or 1/3 cup low-fat egg substitute)

1 tsp fresh or dry dill

1/2 tsp garlic powder

1/4 cup cornflake crumbs

Defrost spinach and squeeze out as much water as possible. Brown chopped onions and scallions in beer, wine, or broth. In medium-sized bowl, mix ricotta, Parmesan, eggs, cornflake crumbs, spinach, onion mixture, dill, and garlic. Melt 1 1/2 tablespoons margarine and get 9 sheets of defrosted phyllo dough ready. Lightly brush both sides of each sheet with margarine. Spread 1/3 spinach mixture evenly in a 9-inch pie plate. Top with 3 sheets of phyllo, lightly brushed on both sides with margarine. Spread another 1/3 of the spinach mixture evenly in pan. Fold all sheets of phyllo hanging out of pan back over the spinach filling and brush with margarine. Lay last 3 sheets of phyllo over the top, lightly brushing both sides with margarine. Spread remaining spinach mixture into pan and fold ends of phyllo back over the top. Brush with remaining margarine. Bake in 400° oven for about 15 to 20 minutes or until golden brown. Makes 6 servings.

Nutritional Analysis: Per Serving (or 1/6 of pie)
Calories 307, Fiber 3 gm, Cholesterol 73 mg, Sodium 725 mg, Percent of calories from: Protein 23%, Carbohydrate 45%, Fat 32% (11 gm)

❖ Special Sauces and Fillings ❖

Carrot Sauce

(Goes great with pasta, chicken, fish, or vegetables)

1 Tbsp butter

1/2 cup low-fat milk

1 1/2 cups finely grated carrots

4 Tbsp low-fat milk

2 tsp cornstarch

3 Tbsp Romano or Parmesan cheese

1/2 tsp oregano

Pepper to taste

Puree grated carrots in blender or food processor with 1/2 cup milk. Melt butter on medium-high heat in Teflon fry pan. Add carrot mixture and let bubble for a minute. In a small dish, mix 2 tsp cornstarch with 2 Tbsp milk. Then add 2 Tbsp more milk. Add to carrot mixture, stir frequently, and let bubble a few minutes more. Reduce heat to simmer. Sprinkle cheese and spices on top, stir, and let simmer several minutes. Makes 3 servings of sauce.

Nutritional Analysis: Per Serving of sauce (Also analyzed with 1 cup pasta noodles per serving)

Calories 112 (285), Fiber 1.6 gm (2 gm), Cholesterol 22 mg, Sodium 165 mg
Percent of calories from: Protein 16% (15%), Carbohydrate 32% (62%), Fat 53% (23%)

Three Cheese Sauce

This sauce can be used to make macaroni and cheese, scalloped potatoes, or cheese-topped broccoli potatoes.

2 Tbsp flour

1 1/4 cup low-fat milk

2 oz part-skim Jarlsberg (or reduced-fat Swiss) cheese, grated

2 1/2 ounces reduced-fat sharp cheddar cheese, grated

2 Tbsp grated Parmesan cheese

1/4 tsp garlic powder, 1/8 tsp pepper

In a small saucepan, blend flour with 2 tablespoons of milk to form a smooth paste. Using a wire whisk, slowly blend in remaining milk until smooth. Simmer over medium heat until nicely thickened. Reduced heat and add all three cheeses, garlic powder, and pepper and stir until well blended and cheese has melted. Remove from heat and use as desired. Makes about 4 servings of sauce.

Nutritional Analysis: Per Serving (numbers in parentheses are for sauce with 1 cup cooked macaroni)
Calories 150 (347), Cholesterol 23 (23) mg, Sodium 266 (267) mg, Percent of calories from: Protein 35% (23%), Carbohydrate 21% (56%), Fat 43% (21%) (7 gm or 8 gm of fat)

Fresh Tomato Cream Sauce

1 Tbsp butter

1 clove garlic, finely minced

1 cup ripe Roma tomatoes (diced) or cherry tomatoes (quartered)

1/4 cup finely diced red bell pepper

1/4 tsp finely crushed dried basil

3/4 cup whole milk

2 tsp flour

2-3 Tbsp grated Parmesan cheese

Pinch or two of nutmeg

About 4 cups cooked fettucini noodles

In nonstick fry pan, melt butter with garlic over medium-high heat. Add tomato pieces and red pepper and let simmer for a few minutes. Sprinkle basil over the top while it's simmering. Add 3/4 cup milk to measuring cup. Mix flour with a tablespoon of the milk and reserve. Pour the remaining milk into the tomato mixture. Then stir in the flour mixture. Keep stirring while it simmers another 2 minutes until cream sauce has thickened. Sprinkle Parmesan cheese and nutmeg on top and stir.

Serve over fettucini noodles. Makes 8 servings.

Nutritional Analysis: Per Serving (served over fettucini noodles)
Calories 327, Fiber 2.5 gm, Cholesterol 22 mg, Sodium 160 mg, Percent of calories from: Protein 15%, Carbohydrate 64%, Fat 21% (8 gm)

Roasted Red Pepper Sauce

(great for pastas and fish)

2 sweet red peppers
3 tsp olive oil
1/2 cup 1% low-fat milk,
1 or 2 cloves garlic, minced
Salt and pepper to taste (optional)
Freshly grated Parmesan cheese (optional)

Turn on broiler. Cut each pepper into quarters and remove inside flesh and seeds.Cut each quarter in half to make 16 strips total. Lay strips on nonstick baking sheet. Brush pepper strips with 1 tsp of oil. Flip to other side and brush with 1 more teaspoon. Broil until top side is nicely browned. Turn pepper strips over to brown other side. Let cool slightly. In food processor, blend pepper strips with milk, garlic, and last teaspoon oil. Salt and pepper to taste. Heat to desired temperature in microwave or on the stove top and pour over pasta or fish. Sprinkle Parmesan cheese over the top if desired. Makes sauce for 4 servings.

Nutritional Analysis: per serving of sauce

Calories 53, Fiber 0.6 gm, Cholesterol 1 mg, Sodium 17 mg, Percent of calories from: Protein 10%, Carbohydrate 28%, Fat 61% (3.7 gm fat). NOTE: Adding the sauce to pasta or fish will lower the percentage of calories from fat.

Tomato-Garlic Sauce

1 to 2 cloves garlic, finely minced

2 tsp olive oil

About 1 1/2 cups coarsely chopped Roma or cherry tomatoes
    (as ripe as possible)

1 Tbsp chopped fresh basil leaves (or 1 tsp dried sweet basil)

1 tsp fresh oregano (or 1/4-1/2 tsp dried)

Ground pepper to taste

2 Tbsp grated Parmesan cheese

Pasta noodles of your choice

While pasta (noodles, ravioli, or tortellini) is boiling, in nonstick fry pan over medium heat, sauté garlic in oil for a minute. Lower heat slightly and add tomato pieces and herbs, and let simmer 3 to 5 minutes until barely thickened. Sprinkle Parmesan over top. Spoon over cooked, drained pasta. Makes 2 servings of sauce.

Nutritional Analysis: Per Serving, including 1 cup of cooked pasta
Calories 294, Fiber 8 gm, Cholesterol 4 mg, Sodium 268 mg, Percent of calories from: Protein 14%, Carbohydrate 62%, Fat 24% (7.7 gms fat)

Super Quick Spaghetti Sauce

1 lb. extra-lean ground beef (less than 13% fat)

1 1/2 cups chopped yellow onion

2 cups grated yellow crookneck squash or zucchini

3 cloves garlic

1 tsp oregano

1 tsp lemon pepper (no-salt blend) or 1/2 tsp black pepper

1 jar spaghetti sauce (32 oz) with 3 grams of fat or less per
    1/2 cup serving

Cooked pasta (about 6 to 9 cups)

Cook beef with garlic, onions, and spices. Then stir in the grated squash for about 5 minutes. Add jar of spaghetti sauce and let simmer for 5 minutes more. Serve over cooked pasta. Makes 6 servings.

Nutritional Analysis: Per Serving, including one cup of cooked pasta
Calories 415, Fiber (not available), Cholesterol 45 mg, Sodium 575 mg, Percent of calories from: Protein 22%, Carbohydrate 58%, Fat 20%

Lite Pesto Sauce

1 cup fresh, shredded basil leaves (tightly packed)

1 clove garlic, finely minced

1 envelope Herb-Ox low-sodium chicken broth (or similar)

1/4 cup 1% (or 2%) milk

1 Tbsp olive oil

1/4 cup Parmesan cheese

2 Tbsp pine nuts or pecan or walnut pieces, toasted (lay nuts in single layer in shallow pan and broil briefly)

In a food processor or blender, briefly chop the first two ingredients. Add the low-sodium chicken broth powder to the milk and mix well. Pour into food processor along with rest of the ingredients. Blend until fairly smooth (about 10 to 15 seconds—stop halfway to scrape the sides of the container). Makes about 2/3 cup pesto sauce.

Nutritional Analysis: Per 2 Tablespoons of Sauce mixed with 1 1/2 cups cooked spaghetti noodles

Calories 360, Fiber 3 gm, Cholesterol 4 mg, Sodium 90 mg, Percent of calories from: Protein 13%, Carbohydrates 69%, Fat 18%

Chicken, Basil, and Baby Carrot Filling

(for pasta or dinner crepes)

  4 chicken breasts (skinned, boned, cut into strips and simmered in 1 cup
    low-sodium chicken broth)
  2 green onions (white and part of green stem), chopped
  1/4 cup fresh parsley, finely chopped
  1 cup lightly packed fresh basil leaves
  1 1/2 cups chopped baby carrots, cooked
  1/3 cup grated Parmesan cheese
  1/4 tsp black pepper

Remove cooked chicken from broth mixture with slotted spoon. Mix all
ingredients together and then process until finely ground. Refrigerate
until needed.

Nutritional Analysis: Per Complete Recipe
Calories 975, Cholesterol 300 mg, Sodium 1095 mg, Percent of calories
from: Fat 21%

❖ Snacks and Desserts ❖

Pear 'N Raisin Crisp

1/2 cup Quaker Oat Bran cereal, uncooked

1 Tbsp packed brown sugar

1/2 tsp cinnamon

1 Tbsp margarine, melted

6 cups thinly sliced pears (about 6)

1/2 cup raisins (or other dried fruit, chopped)

1/4 cup water

1 Tbsp lemon juice

1/4 cup packed brown sugar

2 Tbsp flour

1/2 tsp cinnamon

Heat oven to 375°. Combine cereal, brown sugar, cinnamon, and margarine; mix well. Set aside. Combine pears, raisins, water, and lemon juice in large bowl. Add the remaining ingredients, stirring until pears are evenly coated. Arrange in 8-inch square baking dish; sprinkle oat bran topping evenly over pears. Bake 25 to 30 minutes or until pears are tender. Makes 8 servings.

Nutritional Analysis: Per Serving
Calories 180, Fiber 4 gm, Cholesterol 0 mg, Sodium 20 mg, Percent of calories from: Protein 4%, Carbohydrate 86%, Fat 10%

Oaty Rhubarb Crisp

3 cups fresh rhubarb, sliced (or frozen, unsweetened)

1 1/2 cups fresh strawberry halves (or frozen, unsweetened)

1/3 cup sugar

3 Tbsp flour

1/2 tsp ground cinnamon

1/4 cup orange juice or apple juice

Topping:

1 cup rolled oats

1/3 cup packed brown sugar

1/2 cup flour

1/3 cup shredded coconut

2 Tbsp margarine, melted

1/2 cup low-fat milk

Preheat oven to 350°. In large bowl, stir together granulated sugar, 3 table-spoons flour, and cinnamon. Add rhubarb and strawberries. Pour juice over top and gently toss to mix. Pour into ungreased 8-inch round baking or casserole dish. In small mixing bowl, stir 1/2 cup flour, oats, brown sugar, coconut, and margarine together with a fork. Drizzle milk evenly over the top and stir to coat evenly. Sprinkle topping over filling. Bake for approximately 30 minutes (until rhubarb is tender and topping is golden). Makes 6 generous servings.

Nutritional Analysis: Per Serving

Calories 263, Fiber 5.5 gms, Cholesterol 2 mg, Sodium 63 mg, Percent of calories from: Protein 7%, Carbohydrate 69%, Fat 24% (7 gm)

Lemon Berry Coffee Cake

1 box Pillsbury Plus Lemon Cake mix

1/3 cup light cream cheese (in tub)

2/3 cup nonfat cottage cheese

1 egg

1/3 cup water

3 cups berries (1/2 blueberries and 1/2 raspberries, fresh or frozen)

1/3 cup oat or wheat bran (the flakier the better)

Preheat oven to 350°. In food processor, whip cottage cheese until smooth. Add cream cheese and whip until well blended. On low speed of mixer, blend cheese mixture with cake mix. Reserve about 1 cup of crumb mixture for topping. To the rest, add milk, egg, water, and blend on low speed for one to two minutes. Pour into 8 1/2 x 14-inch pan (use nonstick spray coating generously or lightly grease). Spread berries evenly over the top and press them lightly into batter. Blend bran in with the reserved crumb mixture (use fork to keep it crumbly). Sprinkle it over coffee cake and bake for 35 to 40 minutes. Makes 15 medium servings.

Nutritional Analysis: Per Serving
Calories 179, Fiber 1.5 gm, Cholesterol 20 mg, Sodium 288 mg, Percent of calories from: Protein 10%, Carbohydrate 72%, Fat 18% (3.5 gm)

Frozen Fruit Bars

2 cups summer fruit

1 Tbsp sugar

1 tsp lemon juice

Puree fruit in blender, adding a tablespoon or two of water, if needed. Add sugar (if desired) and lemon juice, and blend. Pour into bar molds or small cups and insert sticks. Freeze until solid. For most fruits, each bar will be less than 50 calories and mostly carbohydrates. This recipe makes 4 bars.

Lemon Strawberry Yogurt Whip

2 1/2 cups strawberries, cut in half

1 6-oz container each Weight Watchers A La Francais lemon and strawberry nonfat yogurt (or similar)

6 oz. Light Cool Whip whipped topping, slightly thawed

Lightly puree strawberries in food processor or blender. Pour into large mixing bowl. Add both yogurt and the whipped topping. Blend with mixer. Gently spoon into separate serving dishes. Refrigerate for one hour before serving and serve within 24 hours for best consistency. Serves 8.

Nutritional Analysis: Per Serving

Calories 125, Fiber 1 gm, Cholesterol 30 mg, Sodium 30 mg, Percent of calories from: Protein 6%, Carbohydrate 62%, Fat 32%

Hot Applesauce Cake

4 Tbsp margarine, softened

2/3 cup sugar

3 egg whites, 1 yolk, lightly beaten

1 cup white flour

1 1/2 cups whole-wheat flour

3/4 cup orange juice

2 cups applesauce, unsweetened

2 tsp baking soda

2 tsp cinnamon *

1 tsp ground cloves *

1 tsp ground allspice *

1/4 tsp nutmeg *

1/4 tsp mace*

  *(or use 4 tsp "pumpkin pie spice" for the spices listed above)

1 cup raisins

1/2 cup walnuts (or other nuts)

Preheat oven to 350°. In large mixing bowl, cream margarine, slowly adding sugar; beat until smooth. Add egg mixture, mix well. Mix dry ingredients together (flours, soda, spices), then add to creamed mixture along with applesauce, orange juice, raisins, and walnuts. Beat until well blended. Pour into nonstick Bundt® (or similar) pan. Bake 40 to 50 minutes (or until toothpick inserted in center comes out clean). Cool 10 minutes, then turn cake out onto plate or rack to cool slightly before serving. If desired, sprinkle cake with powdered sugar. Makes 12 servings.

Nutritional Analysis: Per Serving
Calories 270, Fiber 4 gm, Cholesterol 22 mg, Sodium 200 mg, Percent of calories from: Protein 8%, Carbohydrate 67%, Fat 25%

Cream Sherry Walnut Cake (Using a Mix)

1 yellow cake mix (incomplete)

1 egg and 1 egg white

1 cup cream sherry

1/2 cup walnut pieces

1/3 cup and 2 Tbsp water

1 Tbsp vegetable oil

1/8 cup powdered sugar sifted on top of cake for decoration (optional)

Do not follow directions on cake mix box. Preheat oven to 350°. Add cake mix to a bowl and beat in eggs, sherry, walnuts, water, and oil until smooth. Pour into a nonstick Bundt® or similar-sized pan (or use nonstick cooking spray). Bake for about 35 minutes. Do not over bake! Makes 12 slices.

Nutritional Analysis: Per Slice

Calories 250, Sodium 290 mg, Percent of calories from: Protein 6%, Carbohydrate 63%, Fat 31%

Cream Sherry Walnut Cake (Homemade)

1 3/4 cups flour

1 cup sugar

2 1/2 tsp baking powder

1 tsp salt

1/3 cup butter or margarine, softened

1/2 cup low-fat milk

1 egg

2/3 cup cream sherry

1 tsp vanilla extract

1/2 cup walnuts

In large mixing bowl, mix first four ingredients. Blend in butter and milk for about 1 to 2 minutes at medium speed with mixer. Add eggs, sherry, and vanilla, mixing for 2 minutes more. Scrape bowl constantly. Pour the batter into a Teflon or spray-coated Bundt® or similar-sized cake pan and bake 25 to 35 minutes, until toothpick inserted in center comes out clean. Makes 12 slices.

Nutritional Analysis: Per Slice

Calories 235, Fiber 1 gm, Cholesterol 35 mg, Sodium 300 mg, Percent of calories from: Protein 7%, Carbohydrate 58%, Fat 35%

Chocolate Whiskey Cake
(Using a Mix)

1 box Duncan Hines® Swiss Chocolate Cake mix (or use another chocolate cake mix where they ask you to add the eggs and oil yourself)

3 egg whites, 1 egg yolk, lightly beaten

1/3 cup and 1/4 cup whiskey

3/4 cup water

Preheat oven to 350°. Pour box mix into large mixing bowl. Add whiskey,
egg mixture, and water. Beat well. Pour batter into a nonstick Bundt® pan
(or similar) or use nonstick cooking spray. Bake for about 35 to 40 minutes
(until toothpick inserted in center comes out clean). Lightly sift and sprinkle powdered sugar on top, if you like. Makes 12 servings.

Nutritional Analysis: Per Serving

(Exact values depend on mix used), Percent of calories from: Protein 9%,
Carbohydrate 69%, Fat 22%

Lower-Fat Oatmeal Raisin Cookies

2 1/4 cup flour

1/2 tsp baking soda

1/4 tsp salt

1 cup quick oats (not instant)

1 cup brown sugar

1/2 cup white sugar

1/2 cup butter or margarine

1/2 cup light sour cream

1 Tbsp vanilla extract

1 egg and 2 egg whites

1 1/2 cup raisins

Preheat oven to 300°. In a medium bowl combine first four ingredients and set aside. In mixing bowl, blend sugars than add butter and sour cream and mix at medium speed. Scrape sides and add vanilla and eggs. Continue mixing until light and fluffy.

Turn mixer to low speed and add flour mixture. Stir in raisins. Do not over-mix. Drop by rounded tablespoonfuls or cookie dough scoop onto cookie sheets lightly coated with nonstick spray. Bake about 15 minutes or until desired doneness. You may want to slightly underbake if you perfer your cookies chewy. Makes 36 cookies.

Nutritional Analysis: Per Cookie
Calories 121, Fiber 8 gm, Cholesterol 13 mg, Sodium 64 mg, Percent of calories from: Protein 6%, Carbohydrate 72%, Fat 22% (3 gm fat)

Mint Chocolate Chip Cookies

1/4 cup butter or margarine, softened

1/2 cup reconstituted Butter Buds, chilled

1/2 cup brown sugar

1/2 cup sugar

1 egg and 1 tsp vanilla, beaten

3/4 cup whole wheat flour

3/4 cup white flour

1/2 tsp baking soda

9 oz. mint chocolate chips (or other flavor)

Preheat oven to 350°. Cream butter with sugars and Butter Buds mixture. Add egg and vanilla; beat until fluffy. Combine flours with baking soda, mixing into creamed mixture. Stir in chips. Spoon dough onto a Teflon baking sheet. (Each cookie should be a little less than a tablespoon.) Bake for about 6 to 8 minutes. Watch carefully, taking cookies out of the oven BEFORE they are cooked through, to keep them chewy. Cool on paper towels. Makes about 30 large cookies.

Nutritional Analysis: Per Cookie

Calories 100, Fiber 0.6 gm, Cholesterol 13 mg, Sodium 55 mg, Percent of calories from: Protein 4%, Carbohydrate 60%, Fat 36%

Rum Berry Topping

2 Tbsp Smucker's Low-Sugar Boysenberry Spread (or other flavor)

1 Tbsp rum

Serve over

1 cup vanilla ice milk, low-fat frozen yogurt, or angel food cake

In a saucepan over medium heat, simmer the preserves with the rum for about 5 minutes, stirring frequently. Pour over dessert of choice. Makes 1 serving.

Nutritional Analysis: Per Serving, including ice milk

Calories: 265, Percent of calories from: Protein 8%, Carbohydrate 73%, Fat 19%

Oaty Apricot Tart

Crust:

1 1/2 cup flour

1/2 cup melted butter or margarine

6 to 7 Tbsp cold water

1 Tbsp Molly McButter (or other natural butter-flavored sprinkles) (optional)

Mix butter into flour with fork. Add water, tablespoon by tablespoon, until ingredients start sticking together. Pat into Teflon-coated pie or quiche dish.

Filling:

5 to 6 cups apricots, quartered

2/3 cup sugar

1/2 tsp ground cinnamon

1/4 cup flour

Mix ingredients together and pour evenly into crust shell.

Topping:

1 1/2 cups rolled oats (or low-fat Muesli cereal)

1/2 cup reconstituted Butter Buds, chilled

2 Tbsp melted butter or margarine

Mix topping ingredients and spread evenly over filling.

Bake tart in preheated 425° oven for 15 minutes. Reduce to 350° and bake about 30 minutes longer, until crust browns and the juice bubbles thick around the sides. Makes 12 servings.

Nutritional Analysis: Per Serving
Calories 270, Fiber 3 gm, Cholesterol 27 mg, Sodium 170 mg, Percent of calories from: Protein 7%, Carbohydrate 60%, Fat 33%

Reduced-Fat Blueberry Cheesecake (or other fruit)

Crust:

1 cup flour

1/4 cup margarine, melted

1/4 cup nonfat milk (or low-fat)

Filling:

1 8-oz package Philadelphia Light Cream Cheese (in tub)

1 cup nonfat milk

1/3 cup sugar

1 egg

Topping:

3 cups fresh or frozen blueberries (or other fruit in season, such as strawberries, kiwis, etc.)

2 Tbsp cornstarch

Preheat oven to 350°. Combine crust ingredients and press into 9-inch Teflon pie tin (or use nonstick spray coating). Using a mixer or food processor, blend filling ingredients until smooth. Pour over crust. Bake for about 20 minutes. Meanwhile, in a saucepan, cook blueberries with cornstarch (adding about 1/4 cup water, if necessary), stirring until thickened.

After cheesecake has baked for 20 minutes, pour blueberry mixture evenly over the top and bake for about 20 minutes more (until cream cheese filling has set and crust has lightly browned). Cool. Serves 12.

Nutritional Analysis: Per Serving

Calories 173, Fiber 2 gm, Cholesterol 32 mg, Sodium 170 mg, Percent of calories from: Protein 10%, Carbohydrate 50%, Fat 40%, (Just for comparison's sake: A certain chef's refrigerator cheesecake with blueberries has more than 300 calories per same size slice, with 70% of calories from fat and 133 mg cholesterol!)

Very Berry Smoothie

1 cup fresh or frozen berries (if frozen, thaw slightly)

1/2 cup nonfat milk

3/4 cup low-fat frozen yogurt* (Breyer's, Rhapsody Farms, Yoplait, etc.)
    *Use strawberry or other berry flavors.

Put all three ingredients in a food processor or blender. Blend until smooth. Serves 2.

Nutritional Analysis: Per Serving

Calories 135, Cholesterol 6 mg, Sodium 72 mg, Percent of calories from: Protein 14%, Carbohydrate 70%, Fat 16%

Chapter

The Healthy Happy Hour

You walk in and look around. As you're greeted with a cup of eggnog, you try to remember if this is your third or fourth holiday party this week. You grab a handful of those green and red covered chocolate pieces on your way to talk with a friend. While talking, you nibble on a couple handfuls of potato chips with dip and some crackers and cheese.

Later, when champagne is passed around, you try pieces of the English toffee and fudge sitting on the coffee table, on top of the handfuls of almonds and several toothpicks of speared Vienna sausage that you had somewhere between the chocolate and the champagne. You unsuspectingly walk out of the party carrying a grand total of around 2,200 calories, most of which are from fat.

I'm not suggesting we all roam around each party clasping our calculators and calorie counter booklets, chewing on celery sticks. But we can save ourselves from "the party guilts" by partying with a little extra food wisdom.

The Party Goer's Guide to Healthful Eating

#1. Make better choices

When confronted with the typical party nibblies (nuts, dips, chips, hors d'oeuvres, appetizers, etc.), know which ones are lower in fat and calories and choose these when you can. As far as hors d'oeuvres and appetizers go, stay away from (or limit yourself to a taste of) the cheesy, pastry, eggy, or meaty types. What's left? For other party snacks, you can scrutinize the following table:

	Calories	% Calories from fat
Crackers:		
Ritz, 1	18	48
Wheat Thins, 2	18	36
Saltines, 1	12	25
Bread: *(anything in this category is a better choice)*		
Sourdough, 1/2 slice	35	7
Bagel halves, 1	82	6
Pita bread halves, 1	95	5
Pastries:		
Fruit turnover, 1	340	53
Cream puff with custard, 1	300	54
Danish, 1	275	50
Dips:		
Sour cream, 1/4 cup	123	86
Yogurt, low-fat, 1/4 cup	35	22
Light sour cream, 1/4 cup	90	60
Guacamole, 1/4 cup	93	9
Refried beans, 1/4 cup	75	26
Chips *(1 oz. is about 2 handfuls, depending on the hand)*		
Potato, 1 oz	163	62
Tortilla, 1 oz	139	47
Pretzels, 1 oz	111	11
Cheese twists, 1 oz	153	56
Nuts:		
Peanuts, 1/4 cup	210	73
Almonds, 1/4 cup	246	77

	Calories	% Calories from fat
Spreads, 1/4 cup		
Cheese spread, 1 Tbsp	50	77
Cream cheese, 1 Tbsp	50	90
Sweets:		
Sugar cookie, 1	60	45
Chocolate chip cookie, 1	95	47
Fudge, 1 oz. cube	195	78
English toffee, 1 oz.	195	78
M & M Peanuts, 1 oz.	145	45
Meats/Deli Platter:		
Vienna sausage, 1 small	45	82
Chicken nugget, 1	52	54
Bologna, 1 oz.	90	82
Salami, 1 oz.	70	72
Ham, 1 oz, trimmed of fat	45	33
Turkey breast, fresh, 1 oz. slice	45	19
Cheese, 1 oz. slice	115	74
Brie (or other soft French cheeses), 1 oz	95	8
Fruit Platter (all items in this category are better choices):		
Apple, 1/4 whole	20	5
Pineapple chunks (in juice)	38	1
Melon balls, 1/4 cup	14	6

	Calories	% Calories from fat

Vegetable Platter *(all items in this category are better choices):*

	Calories	% Calories from fat
Broccoli, 1/4 cup	11	10
Cauliflower, 1/4 cup	4	3
Mushrooms, 1/4 cup	4	14
Carrots, 1/4 cup	10	6
Tomato, 1/4 whole	6	6
Green or red pepper, 1/4 cup	12	8
Cucumber, 3 slices	2	5
Celery, 1/4 cup	4	5
Green beans (lightly cooked), 1/4 cup	9	5
Squash strips, 1/4 cup	6	4

#2. Keep portions to a minimum

Remember to eat slowly and enjoy it. The problem with snacks and spreads is that they slowly, without notice, add up over the evening. If you saw what you ate during the party's duration piled all together on a plate, you would probably be shocked. Instead, you can fill a small plate with just a taste of the foods you want to try.

#3. Offer to bring food low in fat

Rolls and nut breads can be a great alternative to the typical high-fat party fare. You can bake many festive (and healthful) breads by following the "Art of Healthful Baking" section in Chapter 6.

A lower fat dip can be made by substituting plain, low-fat yogurt for sour cream or using half light sour cream and half nonfat yogurt. A spinach dip can be made by mixing frozen spinach, minced onion, diced jicama, and spices with yogurt and serving it in a hollowed sourdough bread round (using the cut-out pieces of bread as dippers). Another quick dip can be made by mixing dried soup mix (onion types work well) with plain, low-fat yogurt. However, use only half the amount of soup mix you would normally add to the sour cream. The salty flavor is more pronounced when yogurt is used.

The amount of fat in fancy spreads such as crab or salmon can be reduced by cutting the amount of cream cheese called for in half, by using Philadelphia Light in the tub, or by adding low-fat yogurt, part-skim ricotta cheese, or buttermilk until you get the desired consistency.

You can also offer to bring fruits and vegetable platters to the party so you know there will be something you can nibble on. Lemon or vanilla low-fat yogurt can be used as a dip for fruit.

A special section on cheese and crackers will be found later in this chapter, so read on.

#4. Don't spend all your calories at the bar

Usually we're not thinking too much about "extra" calories or the effect of too much alcohol when we order a double martini or a pitcher of Margaritas. And you certainly aren't thinking about how alcohol calories can easily be converted and stored as fat in the body. Why do you think there's such a thing as a "beer belly?"

Think about what you usually drink during the course of an evening party—or Sunday barbecue, for that matter—and add the damage up, using the table below.

Beverage	Calories
Eggnog, 1 cup	342 (49% from fat)
Wine, 1 cup	259
Champagne, 1 cup	180
Cordials and liqueur, 1 oz	97
Martini, 1 1/2 oz	140
Daiquiri, 3 1/2 oz	125
Other cocktails, 3 1/2 oz	140-180

Beverage	Calories
Beer, 12 oz	145-160
Light beer, 12 oz	100-120
Grapefruit juice, 6 oz	70-80
Orange juice, 6 oz	75-85
Apple cider, 1 cup	110
Fruit punch, 1 cup	132
Sweetened seltzers, 6 oz	70-85
Tonic water, 6 oz	60-70
Assorted soft drinks, 6 oz	70-95

The following items are unsweetened:

Club soda	0
Sparkling water	0
Seltzer	0

But for those of us who DO think about these extra (potential fat) calories, or those who have ever been, or will be, elected "DD" (designated driver) by friends, here are some tips to help you join the party without necessarily downing all the alcohol and extra calories.

If You Prefer Not To Drink ANY Alcohol

- Order or make an orange or cranberry juice spritzer, with half orange or cranberry juice and half club soda. A 12-ounce orange spritzer has 75 calories (from carbohydrate) and about 75 milligrams of vitamin C as a bonus!

- Order club soda or sparkling water (for absolutely no calories) and ask for a twist of lemon or lime to add flavor and festivity to your drink.

- Order decaf or regular coffee (with a dab of whipped cream if you want it to look fancy).

- If you're giving the party, try the Sparkling Punch, Apple Sangria, or Peachy Punch at the end of this chapter. Or make up a punch of your own!

If You Prefer to Drink Less Alcohol

And then there are those of us who just want to drink fewer calories or less alcohol. Call it a security blanket, but we're the people out dancing or at a party who tend to always have a glass in our hand. If you're one of these perpetual sippers, the following tips are especially for you:

- Order a wine spritzer instead of wine or a wine cooler. A wine spritzer is wine with club soda (zero calories in the soda). A wine cooler is wine with regular 7-Up or a similar soda added. A 12-ounce wine cooler will cost you about 170 calories. A wine spritzer will only run about 125 calories. But 12 ounces of wine "straight" will give you twice the alcohol and cost you around 250 calories!

- If you like mixed drinks, try ordering the first one regular and the rest without alcohol. You can usually order a strawberry daiquiri without the alcohol—remember the ones your parents used to order for you before you turned 21? Or you can trade off: one mixed drink, one club soda, one mixed drink, one club soda.

- What about all the veteran beer drinkers? I'm sure there are a bunch out there who poo-poo "light" beers. But what exactly ARE the benefits of saying "Bud Light, please." instead of "I'll have a Budweiser"? Well, the benefits are mostly caloric, since the alcohol content is only slightly lower. Take a look at the table above. What does this mean in terms of a possible evening's worth of beer? If you order three Miller Lites (one of the light beers with the lowest number of calories) instead of three regular beers, for example, you will save yourself about 160 total calories, but only 37 calories from alcohol.

Be aware, though, that some beers are called "light" because of their light color, not their calorie content. If you order a Lowenbrau, and the bartender says, "Light or dark?," he or she means the color. So I suggest if you're interested in drinking a beer lower in calories, get to know which brand you like and order it by name.

Cheese and Crackers

The usual cheese and cracker rendezvous—a popular party cracker such as the "Ritz" or "Trevor Triscuit" meets up with the soft French-looking dish called "Brie." Separately they're dangerous enough, but together? Well, don't expect some enchanted evening—expect a fattening one.

Most of us know that crackers tend to be loaded with fat and salt. But that doesn't mean we never find ourselves buying crackers. A lot of the spreads we cover our crackers with are also high in fat and sodium, and who knows what else.

One ounce of your basic cheddar cheese (about the size of a processed cheese slice) at 115 calories, 74% from fat, lined up with four fatty crackers, such as Ritz (72 calories, 48% from fat) gives you a total of 190 calories, 64% from fat. What did you expect to get when you put two fatty things together? You get even more fat. I don't even want to think about the highly processed types that have so many "other" things added that they have to take on names such as "cheese food." By the way, these squirtable cheeses have 85 to 95 calories per ounce, about 350 mg of sodium, and more than 65% of calories from fat.

If you choose a low-fat cracker, at least you have a running start. Consult Chapter 3 for a list of low-fat crackers (with less than 30% of calories from fat). Now on to the cheese part of the equation.

	Calories	% Calories from fat
Cream cheese, 1 Tbsp	50	90
Sour cream, 1/4 cup	123	86
Light Philadelphia cream cheese, in a tub, 1 Tbsp	30	75
Cheese spread, 1 Tbsp	50	65
Light sour cream, 1/4 cup	90	60
Refried beans, 1/4 cup	75	26
Low-fat yogurt, 1/4 cup	35	22
Low-fat cottage cheese, 1/4 cup	50	20
Nonfat cottage cheese, 1/4 cup	35	<5

It's obvious that the last four are your skinny dip possibilities. Cheese is one of our favorite foods. Unfortunately, cheese IS "fat city!" You can cut your fat per ounce almost in half simply by buying the part-skim (reduced fat) types. Who can refuse an offer like that? To be considered lower in fat, cheese must have 5 grams or less of fat per ounce.

So let's try the revised cheese and cracker rendezvous. Four saltine crackers paired up with one ounce of Laughing Cow Reduced Calorie cheese equals 95 calories, 40% from fat. You could use even less cheese per cracker and lower the percentage of fat even more.

Having a healthy happy hour can be simple if you follow the general party-pointer rules outlined in this chapter. These rules will save you from the party guilt of unwanted extra fat, sodium, and calories, by allowing you to view the party with a little extra food wisdom. One the next several pages you'll find some recipes to help send you on your way.

❖ Entertaining Healthfully ❖
(Low-Fat Recipes Galore!)

Potato Rounds

3 red potatoes, just cooked in the oven
1/3 cup grated sharp cheddar cheese
1/2 cup part-skim ricotta cheese
1/4 cup chopped green onions

Cut the potatoes lengthwise into four rounds each. Mix the remaining ingredients. Spread about 1 tablespoon on each round. Broil for a minute or two or until cheese bubbles. Makes 12 rounds. These can be served as an appetizer on a bed of lettuce or parsley.

Nutritional Analysis: Per Round
Calories 60, Fiber 1 gm, Cholesterol 7 mg, Sodium 33 mg, Percent of calories from: Protein 18%, Carbohydrate 56%, Fat 26%

Chicken Meatballs

14 to 16 ounces of ground chicken breast, uncooked

1 egg white

1/2 cup crackermeal or bread crumbs

1/4 cup green onions, finely chopped

3 Tbsp BBQ sauce

2 cloves garlic, minced

1 Tbsp freshly chopped parsley

Mix all ingredients well in a medium-sized bowl. Shape into 1-inch meatballs. Cook in Teflon skillet over medium heat until brown all around and cooked through. Makes about 30 meatballs, or 5 servings of 6 meatballs each. Serve with spaghetti, as appetizers, with bread as a sandwich, or be creative.

Nutritional Analysis: Per Serving

Calories 160, Fiber 0.5 gm, Cholesterol 50 mg, Sodium 130 mg, Percent of calories from: Protein 55%, Carbohydrate 28%, Fat 17%

Oven-Baked Stuffed Wontons

1 lb boneless, skinless chicken thighs, cut in small pieces and simmered
  in low-sodium chicken broth until cooked throughout

1/3 cup grated carrots

1/3 cup green onion, finely chopped

1 Tbsp low-sodium soy sauce

1/8 tsp pepper

1/2 tsp finely minced fresh ginger

2 tsp dry sherry

1/4 cup Egg Beaters egg substitute

1 (1 lb) package wonton wrappers

In food processor, briefly grind cooked chicken pieces. In bowl, mix
chicken with carrots, onion, soy sauce, pepper, ginger, and sherry until well
blended. Pour Egg Beaters in a separate bowl. To wrap filling in wonton
wrappers, place 1 teaspoon filling in one corner. Fold that corner over the
filling and roll to tuck point under. Moisten the other corners with egg
mixture. Bring these corners downward together and press to seal. Freeze
for later use or bake immediately by spreading 1 to 2 teaspoons oil evenly
on nonstick baking sheet with spatula. Lay wonton on oiled baking sheet.
Flip to other side to coat with oil. Bake in preheated 375° oven until light
brown (10 to 12 minutes). Serve with a variety of sauces. Makes approximately 60 wontons.

Nutritional Analysis: Per wonton using 2 teaspoons oil on pan
Calories 28, Cholesterol 14 mg, Sodium 40 mg, Percent of calories from:
Protein 31%, Carbohydrate 38%, Fat 31%

Baked Chinese Egg Rolls

Egg roll wrappers (available packaged, near the produce section)

1 cup cooked chicken breast, prawns, or tofu, diced

1/4 cup low-sodium chicken broth

4 finely minced scallions

1 1/2 cup slightly cooked cabbage or spinach (boil or steam briefly)

1/2 cup grated carrots

1/2 cup bean sprouts

1/3 cup water chestnuts, chopped

1 clove garlic, minced

1 tsp chopped fresh ginger or 1/4 tsp ground ginger

1 Tbsp "light" soy sauce (or 1 1/2 tsp regular soy sauce)

1 1/2 tsp sesame oil

Preheat oven to 450°. Simmer one cup meat, seafood, or tofu in chicken broth and 1/2 teaspoon sesame oil until cooked throughout. (If using cooked meat, simmer about 3 minutes.) Add more broth if needed. Add everything but the rest of the sesame oil; simmer five minutes more. Let mixture cool about 10 minutes. Place 1/4 cup filling in a rectangular shape on the center of each egg-roll wrapper and fold up envelope style (first each of the ends, then the bottom and top flaps). Seal the last flap with a paste made of 1 tablespoon flour and 2 tablespoons cold water. Place on a Teflon baking sheet, greased with one teaspoon sesame oil. (You can spread it evenly with a plastic spatula.) Flip egg rolls over once to coat each side with a bit of oil. Bake for five minutes more, or until brown, then turn rolls over and bake for five minutes more, again until brown. Makes 8 egg rolls. Serve with Chinese mustard or sweet and sour sauce.

Nutritional Analysis: Per Egg Roll (not including sauce), NOTE: This recipe was analyzed using prawns as the meat item.

Calories 70, Fiber 2 gm, Cholesterol 40 mg, Sodium 370 mg, Percent of calories from: Protein 34%, Carbohydrate 48%, Fat 18%

Broccoli Quiche Squares

1 lb broccoli (about 2 sections) steamed or microwaved until barely cooked, then chopped into small pieces

4 Tbsp white flour

2 eggs

2 oz part-skim mozzarella, grated (or other part-skim cheese)

1/4 cup chopped parsley

1/2 tsp dried oregano

1/2 tsp dried basil

1 cup low-fat cottage cheese

1 cup part-skim ricotta cheese

1 Tbsp lemon juice

1/4 tsp pepper

1/3 cup Italian-style bread crumbs (other types can be used)

Whip flour with beaten eggs. Add broccoli and the remaining ingredients, except bread crumbs, mixing gently. Coat a 9-inch square pan with cooking spray (or use a nonstick pan). Pour in the mixture. Sprinkle bread crumbs on top. Bake 35 to 40 minutes. Cool for a few minutes. Cut into 25 squares (5 rows in each direction).

Nutritional Analysis: Per Square
Calories 45, Fiber 1 gm, Cholesterol 25 mg, Sodium 120 mg, Percent of calories from: Protein 35%, Carbohydrate 29%, Fat 36%

Pesto Cheese Rounds

4 bread rolls (about 8 oz altogether)

2 Tbsp Pesto for Pasta (frozen pesto)

   (or use some other pesto, but drain off some of the oil)

4 oz part-skim mozzarella cheese, grated

Preheat oven to 400°. Cut rolls in half, then remove a little of the inside bread (to make a cavity). Melt pesto, if frozen. Spread pesto evenly on the 8 halves. Sprinkle each half with grated cheese. Bake for about 4 minutes. Turn oven to broil, placing rolls about 3 inches from the broiler unit, and broil about one minute, watching carefully. Makes 8 appetizer servings.

Nutritional Analysis: Per Serving

Calories 120, Cholesterol 9 mg, Sodium, not available, Percent of calories from: Protein 21%, Carbohydrate 57%, Fat 22%

Dried Tomato
and Cheese Appetizers

16 cracker rounds or squares (use low-fat crackers, such as saltines, melba rounds, etc.)

2 1/2 ounces (about 1/2 cup) chevre (fresh goat cheese)

16 slices of dried tomatoes (if packed in oil, drain WELL)

Garnish of fresh basil leaves, shredded or chopped

Spread one tablespoon of cheese over two crackers. Top with two slices of dried tomato. Garnish with fresh basil pieces. Makes 8 appetizers of 2 crackers each.

Nutritional Analysis: Per 2 Crackers

Calories 60, Fiber 1 gm, Cholesterol 8 mg, Sodium 90 mg, Percent of calories from: Protein 19%, Carbohydrate 46%, Fat 35%

Mini Pizzas

2 (11-ounce) cans Pillsbury Soft Breadsticks
25 Tbsp Low-fat Spaghetti Sauce
1 cup part-skim mozzarella cheese, grated
1 cup Kraft Light & Natural cheddar cheese, grated
1/2 cup grated Parmesan cheese
1/2 cup finely chopped sun-dried tomatoes
1/2 cup finely chopped colorful vegetables
  (such as green pepper, carrots, etc.)

Preheat oven to 375°. Mix cheeses together in a bowl. Open can of breadstick dough. Roll out strips in one piece, on lightly floured surface, to form one large rectangle. Using a round cookie cutter, 2 1/2 inches wide, cut about 13 pizza rounds per can. Place dough rounds on a Teflon cookie sheet. Top each round with 1 tablespoon spaghetti sauce. Evenly sprinkle with cheese mixture and garnish each round with your finely chopped vegetables (your choice). Bake until crust is lightly browned and cheese bubbled (about 10 to 15 minutes, but watch carefully). Makes 26 mini pizzas.

Nutritional Analysis: Per Mini Pizza
Calories 90, Cholesterol 8 mg, Sodium 270 mg, Percent of calories from: Protein 22%, Carbohydrate 47%, Fat 31%

Chicken Apple Champagne Sausages

2 small to medium red or green apples, cored and grated
1 onion, finely chopped
1 cup cracker meal or bread crumbs
1/2 cup dry champagne or sparkling dry white wine
1 lb. ground chicken or turkey breast
1/8 tsp pepper
1/2 tsp curry powder (optional)

Cook the apple and onion in a nonstick skillet over low heat, covered, until they are soft (about 4 minutes). Combine cracker meal and champagne in a bowl. Add the ground chicken, pepper, curry, if desired, and apple-onion mixture and mix well with spoon. Shape sausage meat into 20 to 24 patties about 1/2 inch thick. Heat a nonstick skillet over medium heat and cook the patties until the undersides are brown. Then turn patties over and brown other side (about 5 minutes total). Makes 8 servings. Serve with brunch or as appetizers.

Nutritional Analysis: Per Serving
Calories 150, Fiber 1.5 gm, Cholesterol 35 mg, Sodium 35 mg, Percent of calories from: Protein 43%, Carbohydrate 46%, Fat 11%

❖ Dips and Spreads ❖

Salmon Spread

7 1/2 ounces of freshly cooked salmon or smoked salmon (or use canned
   salmon, but pick out pieces of skin and bone)

1/2 cup Light Philadelphia cream cheese (in tub)

1/4 cup part-skim ricotta cheese

1/3 cup (heaped) jicama or water chestnuts, finely chopped

1/4 cup white onion, finely chopped

1 Tbsp parsley flakes

1/2 tsp black pepper

1 loaf French bread, cut into 16 slices

Mix all ingredients, except bread, VERY BRIEFLY, in food processor or
blender. Stir the mixture around and briefly blend again if necessary.
Keep well chilled. (You can make this a day before you need it.) Spread
one tablespoon of spread on each 1/2 slice of bread. (Makes about 2 cups
of spread.)

Nutritional Analysis: Per Serving (1/2 slice of bread)

Calories 68, Sodium 140 mg, Cholesterol, not available, Percent of calories
from: Protein 20%, Carbohydrate 60%, Fat 20%

Crab Spread

6 oz fresh crab, shredded

1/2 cup Philadelphia Light cream cheese, at room temperature

1/4 cup low-fat yogurt, plain

1/3 cup chopped water chestnuts or jicama

1 Tbsp onion flakes

1 Tbsp parsley flakes

1/2 tsp pepper

1/8 tsp salt

1 loaf French bread or low-fat crackers

Mix crab, cream cheese, yogurt, and seasonings together. Add water chestnuts. Makes about 2 cups of spread. Spread about one tablespoon of crab mixture on each half slice of French bread.

Nutritional Analysis: Per 1/2 Slice of Bread Serving

Calories 65, Fiber 0.1 gm, Cholesterol 6 mg, Sodium 165 mg, Percent of calories from: Protein 18%, Carbohydrate 62%, Fat 20%

Almost Fat-Free
Creamy Dip

1 small envelope Hidden Valley Ranch "Lite" dressing mix
1 1/2 cup non-fat milk
1/2 cup non-fat plain yogurt
1 tsp reduced-calorie mayonnaise

Mix the ingredients in a blender or food processor. Makes about two cups of dip or dressing.

Nutritional Analysis: Per 2 Tablespoons
Calories 20, Cholesterol 1 mg, Sodium 210 mg, Percent of calories from:
Protein 21%, Carbohydrate 72%, Fat 7%

Spinach Dip
(in Sourdough Round)

1 sourdough bread loaf, round

1/2 cup nonfat mayonnaise

1/2 cup light mayonnaise

1 cup light sour cream (i.e., Land O'Lakes 2/3rds less fat)

1 5-oz can sliced water chestnuts, drained and chopped

5 green onions, white and green part, chopped

1 package leek, onion or vegetable soup mix (i.e., Knorr Soup Mix)

1 10-oz package frozen chopped spinach (squeeze out excess water)

Cut out top and center portion of sourdough round to make a bowl for the spinach dip. Cut the remaining bread into cubes for dipping. In medium sized bowl, blend mayonnaises, and sour cream with soup mix powder. Mix in water chestnuts, onions, and well drained spinach. Spread into sourdough bowl. Serve with bread cubes. Makes 12 appetizer servings.

Nutritional Analysis: Per Serving

Calories 200, Fiber 2 gm, Sodium approx. 600 mg, Percent of calories from: Protein 11%, Carbohydrate 62%, Fat 27% (6 gm fat)

Crab Mold

8 ounces crab meat (fresh, frozen, or canned, drained well)
1 can Campbell's Healthy Request Cream of Mushroom Soup
1 package Knox plain, unflavored gelatin
4 ounces Philadelphia light cream cheese (in tub)
4 ounces Philadelphia Free cream cheese
1/2 cup fat-free mayonnaise or miracle whip
1/2 cup light mayonnaise
1/2 cup chopped green onions (green and white sections)
1 cup finely chopped celery

Heat concentrated cream of mushroom soup in medium saucepan over medium-low heat. Add gelatin and cream cheeses and let come to gentle boil. Let boil, stirring frequently, until cream cheese melts and gelatin dissolves. Remove from heat. Stir in mayonnaises, crab, green onions and celery. Spread into 1 quart mold or larger, and refrigerate until set. Serve with thinly sliced French or sourdough baggette, water crackers, or other low-fat crackers. Makes 16 spread servings.

Nutritional Analysis: Per Serving (spread only)
Calories 80, Cholesterol 16 mg, Sodium 365 mg, Percent of calories from: Protein 30%, Carbohydrate 24%, Fat 46% (4 gm fat)

Fresh-Mex Bean Dip

16 oz can Rosarita No-fat refried beans

1/2 package taco mix

2 ounces diced green chilies (canned)

3 small green onions, chopped

2 large tomatoes, chopped

4 ounces grated reduced-fat cheese (i.e., Cracker Barrel Light Sharp Cheddar and Light Monterey Jack)

2 ounces chopped olives

1/2 cup light sour cream

Optional:

1/2 cup guacamole (made with nonfat sour cream)

Mix refried beans with taco mix and green chilies. Spread on bottom 9 x 9" baking dish. Spread with sour cream or optional guacamole. Then sprinkle chopped olives, onions, and tomatoes over the top. Top with grated cheese. Serve with "baked" or regular tortilla chips. Makes 8 appetizer servings.

Nutritional Analysis: Per Serving (not including chips)

Calories 97, Fiber 4 gm, Cholesterol 8 mg, Sodium approx. 500 mg (depending on the taco seasoning), Percent of calories from: Protein 28%, Carbohydrate 47%, Fat 25% (3 gm fat)

❖ Party Drinks ❖

Banana Eggnog

2 ripe bananas

1/2 cup nonfat egg substitute

1 tsp sugar

2 cups chilled skim milk

2 tsp vanilla extract

ground nutmeg

Peel and mash bananas. Add egg and sugar and blend until smooth. Add milk and vanilla and continue to mix until just combined. To serve, pour into chilled glasses and sprinkle with nutmeg. Makes 4 servings.

Nutritional Analysis: Per Serving

Calories 84, Fiber 0.5 gm, Cholesterol 2.5 mg, Sodium 92 mg, Percent of calories from: Protein 30%, Carbohydrate 65%, Fat 5%

Apple Sangria

1 orange and 1 lemon, cut into slices

Juice of one lemon

1 cup orange juice

1/4 tsp cinnamon

1 (6 oz) can frozen apple juice concentrate, thawed

1 (25 oz) bottle sparkling apple cider, well chilled

2 cups (or more) sparkling water or club soda

Place orange and lemon slices in a large pitcher. Sprinkle with cinnamon.
Blend in rest of ingredients, adding the sparkling water at the end to taste.
Serves 8.

Nutritional Analysis: Per Serving

Calories 90, Fiber 0.6 mg, Sodium 10 mg, Percent of calories from:
Protein 2%, Carbohydrate 96%, Fat 2%

Sparkling Punch

2 cups orange juice

3 Tbsp lemon juice (juice of one lemon)

6 oz unsweetened pineapple juice

1 cup unsweetened apple juice

12 oz sparkling mineral water or club soda

In a large pitcher, combine the fruit juices and sparkling water. Pour over
ice. Makes about four 10-ounce servings.

Nutritional Analysis: Per 10-ounce Serving

Calories 110, Fiber 1 gm, Sodium 10 mg, Percent of calories from: Protein
4%, Carbohydrate 93%, Fat 3%

Peachy Punch

2 large frozen sliced peaches, partially thawed

12 oz. apricot nectar, chilled

1/4 cup lime juice

1/4 tsp almond extract

32 oz club soda or sparkling mineral water

Place peaches in food processor or blender. With food processor running, add nectar to form a puree. Add lime juice and extract. Add this to a punch bowl, straining first if you want. Gradually mix in club soda to taste. Makes about 10 servings.

Nutritional Analysis: Per Serving

Calories 60, Fiber 2.5 gm, Sodium 6 mg, Percent of calories from: Protein 5%, Carbohydrate 94%, Fat 1%

Festive Not Fattening: Favorite Holiday Recipes

During the holidays we're in a perpetual state of "celebration." But it's not the festivities that get us into trouble as much as it is our "eat-now-pay-later" splurge mentality.

We barely recover from the Halloween-inspired "little candy bar syndrome" (when we can't resist eating those cute mini-sized candies)...and before we know it we're sitting down to a Thanksgiving feast. From then on it's parties, parties, and more parties, straight through Christmas and onto New Year's. So what we're really talking about is a three-month stint of splurging! No wonder we all start the new year 10 pounds heavier.

The answer? A month supply or Dexatrim tablets in your Christmas stocking? Or fasting until Valentines day? Of course not. Prevent those extra 10 from creeping on in the first place. The trick is eating the same healthful way all year long. Of course it always helps to plan a good defense during the holidays to keep from overeating too terribly. This is no time for the little extras that add up to BIG calories and fat, like buttering slices of nut bread or dipping chips. The overeating experts also warn not to fast and feast. You are more likely not to gorge yourself on high fat and calorie party foods if you continue eating regular meals.

And yes, you CAN fit low-fat, lower calorie eating into your holiday plans—especially if you happen to be the one wearing the apron. Often huge reductions in calories and fat can be made in your favorite holiday recipes simply by using a lower fat version of the ingredients called for. We're not talking about doing anything fancy here, folks. How hard can it be to buy light cream cheese and light sour cream instead of regular for your mini cheesecakes or to grab the evaporated skim milk instead of cream for your pumpkin pie? These are changes anyone can make in their recipes. Here are some more ideas on lower fat substitutes for the higher fat ingredients in your favorite holiday recipes:

Count your Savings!

In addition to counting our blessings this Thanksgiving lets treat our lower fat ingredient substitutions to a little mathematical magic, too.

- Most pumpkin pie recipes call for at least 1 cup of cream or evaporated whole milk and 2 eggs. Using evaporated skim milk and 3 egg whites will save you about 220 calories and 30 to 38 grams of fat (and up to 90 milligrams of cholesterol.

- Buying brown and serve rolls instead of the higher fat crescent type rolls will save you from 1,100 extra calories and about 100 grams of fat per dozen.

- Using a combination of nonfat cottage cheese (whipped in food processor) and light cream cheese in your holiday dips or spreads will save you 480 calories and 59 grams of fat per cup of regular cream cheese normally called for.

- Using part-skim sharp cheddar (like Kraft® Light n' Natural sharp cheddar) and light cream cheese, and adding none of the butter or nuts usually called for in your typical holiday cheese log or ball will save 755 calories and 84 grams of fat! (You can also roll your log in cracker crumbs or toasted oats instead of nuts).

- Making your famous onion dip with Land O'Lakes light sour cream and reduced-calorie mayonnaise will save you around 500 calories and 64 grams of fat per cup of dip.

The Holiday Cookie Tray

I don't know about you, but I may be able to forsake the gooey fudge and creamy eggnog during the holidays (all in the line of 'weight watching' duty), but I can only pass by the mesmerizing holiday cookie tray once or twice before my fingers do the walking and select a couple to sample...so many colors and flavors to choose from. Peppermint or Cranberry Red, Dark Molasses Brown, Eggnog yellow, citrus orange, and on and on.

As a chronic recipe modifier, take my word for it. Cookies are a nutritionist's nightmare! Don't get me wrong, I love a challenge. But cookies take the cake (pardon the pun). Cookies are basically a mixture of fat, sugar and flour. Take the fat out and what have you got? Sweet bread (which tastes a might bit different than a cookie!)

Lowering the fat in cookies isn't impossible. It's just that you can usually only lower the butter, margarine, or shortening by 1/3 without anyone noticing. Cut the fat in half, and you're going to hear a few choice words from the peanut gallery. That, and you're bound to end up with a tray full of cookies at the end of the holidays. But I'm not one to scare this easily! So, giving it every ounce of experience and where-with-all I had, I set out to cut the fat in half in four fabulous holiday favorites. But that's not all, I took them to the streets...I taste tested these cookies on normal people (people who don't make a living as a nutritionist and people who aren't related to or don't live with a nutritionist), because people who are highly motivated toward health tend to be a little more forgiving in the flavor department. How many of these four survived the taste test? Would you believe all of them?

Peppermint Pinwheel Cookies

1/3 cup + 2 Tbsp evaporated skim milk

1/2 cup margarine or butter, softened

3 cups all-purpose flour

1 cup sugar

1 egg

1 1/2 tsp vanilla extract

1/2 tsp baking soda

1/4 tsp salt

1 tsp peppermint extract

1/2 tsp red food coloring

In medium-large mixing bowl, beat 1/3 cup evaporated skim milk and butter with electric mixer on medium speed until softened (30 seconds). Add half of the flour, and all the sugar, egg, 2 Tbsp evaporated milk, vanilla, baking soda, and salt to the butter mixture. Beat till completely combined. Beat or stir in remaining flour. Divide dough in half. To one portion stir in peppermint extract and food coloring. Refrigerate at least 4 hours.

To shape dough: between two sheets of waxed paper, roll each portion into a 12 x 11-inch rectangle (or close). Use a little bit of flour if dough seems to stick to roller or waxed paper. Remove top sheets of waxed paper from both doughs. Lay plain dough on top of pink (with waxed paper now on the bottom and on top. Peel off top sheet and roll up from the longest side like a jelly-roll, removing bottom sheet of waxed paper as you go.

With a sharp serrated knife, cut dough into 1/4-inch thick slices. Place on ungreased nonstick cookie sheet. Bake in a 375° oven for 8 to 10 minutes. Edges should be firm and bottoms lightly brown. Remove cookies from pan immediately and let cool on wire rack or plate. Makes 48 cookies.

Nutritional Analysis: Per Cookie

Calories 77, Fiber 0.25 gm, Cholesterol 5 mg, Sodium 58 mg, Percent of calories from: Protein 7%, Carbohydrate 64%, Fat 29% (2.5 gm fat), Original cookie recipe has 100 calories, 46% calories from fat (5 gm), and 40 mg cholesterol.

Oatmeal Scotchies

1 1/2 cup all-purpose flour
(was 1 1/4 cup in original recipe)
1 tsp soda
1/2 tsp salt
1/2 tsp cinnamon
1/2 cup nonfat cottage cheese whipped in food processor with
2 Tbsp evaporated skim milk (wasn't in original recipe)
1/2 cup butter, softened (was 1 cup in original recipe)
2/3 cup sugar (was 3/4 cup)
2/3 cup firmly packed brown sugar (was 3/4 cup)
1 egg with 1/4 cup egg substitute or 2 egg whites (was 2 eggs)
1 tsp vanilla extract
3 cups quick or old-fashioned oats, uncooked
1 1/4 to 1 1/2 cups (7.5 to 9 oz) Nestle's Toll House® butterscotch-fla-
vored morsels (was 12 oz in original recipe)

Preheat oven to 375°. In small bowl, combine flour, baking soda, salt and
cinnamon and set aside. In large mixing bowl, beat butter, nonfat cottage
cheese mixture, sugars, egg and egg substitute, and vanilla extract until
creamy. Gradually beat in flour mixture. Stir in oats and butterscotch chips.
Drop by tablespoonfuls onto ungreased cookie sheets. Bake 8 to 10 minutes. Makes about 48 cookies.

Nutritional Analysis: Per Cookie (using 1 1/4 cup butterscotch morsels)
Calories 100, Fiber 0.7 gm, Sodium 78 mg, Percent of calories from:
Protein 8%, Carbohydrate 61%, Fat 31% (3.5 gm fat). Original recipe has
133 calories and 43% of calories from fat (6.5 gm fat).

Molasses Spice Leaves
(or trees)

1/3 cup walnuts or pecans (was 1/2 cup in original recipe)

2 cups flour

1/4 cup sugar

1/4 cup butter, softened (was 1/2 cup in original recipe)

1/4 cup nonfat plain yogurt (to replace the 1/4 butter we deleted)

1/2 cup firmly packed brown sugar

2 tsp vanilla extract

1/4 cup no-sulphur molasses

1 egg

1/2 tsp ground cardamom

1/2 tsp ground ginger

1/2 tsp ground allspice

1/2 tsp ground cinnamon

1/2 tsp baking soda

Optional icing: 1 1/2 cups powdered sugar beaten with 1 egg white until smooth. Spoon icing into pastry bag with tip of your choice. Decorate tops of cookies with icing and silver balls, if desired.

Finely grind walnuts in food processor. Add 1/3 cup flour and 1/4 cup sugar and blend to powder. Using mixer, cream butter with brown sugar and vanilla in large bowl until blended and somewhat fluffy. Beat in molasses and the egg. Mix remaining 1 3/4 cup flour with nut mixture, spices, and baking soda. Stir into butter mixture. Dough will be sticky. Divide dough in half. Flatten each half into a 1/2-inch thick patty. Wrap each tightly in plastic wrap and refrigerate 4 hours or overnight.

To roll: Preheat oven to 350°. On heavily floured surface, roll 1 of the dough patties out until no more than 1/4-inch thick. Cut out cookies using a 3-inch leaf or tree cookie cutter. Transfer cookies to nonstick baking sheet. Gather scraps and chill another 15 to 30 minutes. Reroll and cut out cookies. Bake cookies until golden (about 8 minutes). Remove from pan immediately and cool on plate or rack.

NOTE: These cookies can be frozen or refrigerated in an airtight container up to 2 weeks!

Nutritional Analysis: Per Cookie

Calories 68, Cholesterol 9 mg, Sodium 29 mg, Percent of calories from: Protein 7%, Carbohydrate 65%, Fat 28% (2 gm fat). Icing will add about 15 calories (mostly carbohydrate) per cookie. The original recipe (without icing) has 82 calories with 40% calories from fat (4 gm).

Holiday Thumbprint Cookies

1 cup all-purpose flour

1/8 tsp salt

1/4 cup butter, softened (was 1/2 cup in original recipe)

2 Tbsp Light cream cheese, in tub (wasn't in original recipe)

2 Tbsp evaporated skim milk (wasn't in original recipe)

1/3 cup sugar

1 egg yolk

1 tsp vanilla extract

1/2 cup walnut or hazelnuts coarsely ground (was 3/4 cup)

Raspberry preserves, approx. 12 tsp (use the lower sugar types if desired)

Preheat oven to 350°. Lay walnut pieces in single layer on pie tin (or similar) and heat in oven until just lightly brown (about 4 minutes), watch carefully. Combine flour and salt in small bowl. In medium-large mixing bowl, cream butter, light cream cheese and evaporated milk until smooth. Add sugar and beat until blended. Mix in yolk and vanilla. Add dry ingredients and nut and mix just until blended. Dough will be sticky.

Refrigerate until dough is a little easier to handle (about 30 minutes). Form dough with hands into 1-inch balls. Place on ungreased cookie sheet. Press thumb into the center of each cookie. Bake 10 minutes. Use a knife to fill each center with the preserve of your choice. Bake another 8 to 10 minutes or until cookies begin to turn light brown. Remove from pan immediately and let cool on rack or plate. Makes 2 dozen delicious cookies!

Nutritional Analysis: Per Cookie (using regular-calorie preserves)
Calories 77, Fiber 0.3 gm, Cholesterol 14 mg, Sodium 39 mg, Percent of calories from: Protein 8%, Carbohydrate 50%, Fat 42% (3.5 gm fat) . Original recipe has 99 calories with 56% calories from fat (6.3 gm fat).

Holiday Stuffing

Unless you want to feel like you're the goose that was cooked and stuffed this Thanksgiving holiday, you are probably already conspiring to lighten up the traditional feast. My advice? Three words: start with stuffing. Stuffing is one of the fattiest foods on the Thanksgiving dinner table. Don't get me wrong—it's also one of the best! So don't give" it up..."lighten" it up!

First thing to do is don't "stuff" your stuffing into the big bird. Picture a large ladle, full of turkey fat, dripping into your fresh, savory stuffing. Need I remind you, you will already be getting a stiff dose of turkey drippings with the gravy.

The next save-the-stuffing step is to cut the margarine/butter from the usual 1/2 stick (4 Tbsp) to only one tablespoon. One tablespoon is all you really need to sauté the celery and onions in, and you will be adding chicken broth to moisten the dry bread flakes or cubes anyway. So just add a little more broth to replace the moistening value of the 3 Tbsp of fat we've taken out. You will hardly notice the difference.

There are two other ways extra fat can creep into your stuffing: from the sausage and from the nuts you might be tempted to add. For the recipe we've lightened-up below, we simply switched to Jimmy Dean "Light" sausage (or similar turkey or turkey-blend sausage). And of all the nuts you can add, roasted or braised chestnuts are by far the lowest in fat and probably the most festive and seasonal of all. One cup of shelled chestnuts add 350 calories and only 3 grams of fat, compared to pecans or walnuts which add about 780 calories and 76 grams of fat!

Now for the giblets and gizzards some stuffing recipes tell you saute with the onions. Organ meats not only contain fat, they are infested with incredible amounts of cholesterol. So it might be best to put those funny looking things back in the bag they came in.

Now take a look at how I made over a basic sausage stuffing recipe:

Apple-Sausage Bread
Stuffing

2 Tbsp diet margarine
2 large tart apples, diced
6 oz. Light Jimmy Dean Sausage
1/4 tsp ground cinnamon
1/2 tsp ground thyme
1/2 tsp diet margarine
1 1/2 cups low-sodium chicken broth
4 cups Pepperidge Farm® Herb Seasoned Stuffing (about 8 oz.)

In a large nonstick frying pan or Dutch oven, brown sausage, breaking it up
into bite-sized bits. Remove the sausage with a slotted spoon and set aside.
In the same pan, melt 2 tablespoons of diet margarine over medium heat.
Add the diced apples and cook, stirring frequently, until the apple pieces
are fairly tender and browned. Add in sausage bits, cinnamon, and thyme.

In a separate Dutch oven or large saucepan, melt 1/2 tablespoon of diet
margarine. Pour in chicken broth and let simmer until just boiling. Turn off
heat. Stir in herb-seasoned stuffing and apple-sausage mixture. Cover and
let sit for 15 minutes or so. Makes 8 side servings.

Nutritional Analysis: Per Serving
Calories 215, Fiber 1.5 gm, Cholesterol 19 mg, Sodium 200 mg, Percent of
calories from: Protein 13%, Carbohydrate 56%, Fat 32% (7.5 gm fat with
sausage, 4 gm fat without sausage)

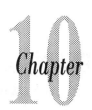

Cutting Fat Forever

Well, you've made it this far, so I know you know what you need to know to cut the fat in your diet—for now. Why not forever? Because forever is a long time. And in order for you to voluntarily eat the low-fat way for the rest of your life, a few things need to happen.

You need to not only believe that a low-fat diet will improve your overall health and reduce your risk of heart disease and cancer, but you have to really want this for yourself. Unfortunately for many people, something drastic (like a death in the family or an extremely high serum cholesterol test result) has to scare them into realizing it can happen to them. Time and time again I've seen a thankfully nonfatal heart attack transform a patient into someone filled with conviction and discipline.

Secondly, it has to be easy. I've said it before, and I'll say it one more time: Few people are willing (or able, for that matter) to give up their busy, on-the-go lifestyle. So for the new, low-fat way of eating to last beyond a month of mere good intentions, it has to fit into your present way of life. And as luck would have it, you have just been shown how the low-fat eating guidelines can be easily incorporated into every eating experience, from fast food to quick meals at home, simply by making smarter choices. You don't necessarily need to change where or how you eat, just change what you eat.

Of course, in order for anything to last forever (including low-fat eating), you have to love it. You have to actually enjoy eating food lower in fat. No one is going to voluntarily sentence themselves to a life of bland, boring food. But now you know that low-fat eating can include most of America's favorite foods, such as pizza, lasagna, and tacos.

Once you've had some practice, ordinary fatty food may even seem very unappealing to you. To me, there is nothing appetizing about finding oil floating around in the bottom of a pasta salad or watching mayonnaise turn yellow on a summer picnic, or being able to see all the white fat globules, clear as day, in fatty sausage or a slice of salami. I don't even like the feeling of immobilizing "fullness" that unavoidably arrives after a cream-laden French or Italian dinner. Maybe someday soon you'll feel the same.

Once You're Living a Life Low in Fat

Once you are really and truly living a life low in fat (less than 30 percent of calories from fat), there are better fats you can choose that might help lower your serum cholesterol levels even further. Generally the "better fats" are the less saturated fats. Perhaps you've heard the terms "polyunsaturated fats" or "monounsaturated fats."

Fats are composed of fatty acids that can either be a monounsaturated fatty acid (with one unsaturated chemical bond), polyunsaturated fatty acid (with more than one unsaturated chemical bond), or a saturated fatty acid (with all chemical bonds saturated). So the "less saturated" fats are your mono- and polyunsaturated fats.

But don't get sucked into the good fat, bad fat sales pitch, either. Remember: All fat in excess of 30 percent of calories from fat is probably bad for your overall health.

The Great Vegetable-Oil Wars

Americans are fickle when it comes to vegetable oils. Five years ago, the magical oil was safflower because it was "high in polyunsaturates." A year ago, it was olive oil because monounsaturated fats were the fatty acid of choice. Today, canola oil has hit the spotlight because it's the oil "lowest in saturated fat" while tropical oils are on the outs because they're high in saturated fat.

While "fat" on our bodies or in our food has clearly become the big "No No" of the nineties, somehow vegetable oil has managed to surface unscathed in the eyes of the public and the media. We all seem to be forgetting that oil is 100 percent fat! And that goes for all "Light" and "No Cholesterol" oils, too. Why is it so easy for us to get sold on the oil of the week? Because people desperately want to believe fats are okay as long as they're using the right fat.

Sorry, but if reducing your risk for obesity and some cancers happens to be a concern, then the low-fat diet, which means a diet low in vegetable oils, too, is the ONLY way to go. Recent animal studies have shown that a diet high in polyunsaturated fats may be linked to certain cancers. And we now know from research that fat calories are more likely than carbohydrate calories to turn into body fat.

But within a low-fat diet (with less than 30 percent of total calories from fat), some fats are better than others. It's the polyunsaturated and monounsaturated fats that are preferred over saturated fats. This is mainly because saturated fats are potent raisers of blood cholesterol levels, even more so than cholesterol-containing foods.

Now for the tricky part. Most vegetable oils are naturally unsaturated (either high in polyunsaturates or monounsaturates), except for the tropical oils (coconut, cocoa butter, palm, and palm kernel oil), which are extremely high in saturated fats. Tropical oils are commonly used in processed foods, such as cookies, cakes, pastries, and nondairy creamers, because they're less expensive and have a longer shelf life. Some food companies also say people prefer the way these oils taste.

Other vegetable oils (corn, soy, and sunflower) can also become uncharacteristically saturated by undergoing a solidifying process called "hydrogenation." This occurs when margarines or shortenings are made. More of their beneficial unsaturated fats then become saturated.

Are some oils absorbed into food less readily than others during frying? (This would mean less fat actually gets into your bloodstream.) Despite commercials advertising otherwise, a *Consumer Reports* study several years back showed all oils are absorbed more or less the same.

This vegetable oil stuff is such a hot topic that I recently received information on yet another brand new oil. This one says it's the best because it has the "highest monounsaturated fat content." It's called Trisun oil and is only being marketed to food processors so far. So don't be surprised to see this unusual oil listed as an ingredient on your box of cereal or crackers in the near future.

True, it wins the contest for the most monounsaturated fat, but it doesn't win the lowest in saturated fat award. That title still belongs to the other unusual sounding oil, canola.

Is it true some oils shouldn't be used at higher temperatures, such as for deep frying or stir-frying? Yes, certain oils have a lower smoke point (the temperature at which the oil starts to foam or smoke). Smoking or foaming is an indication that oxidation and chemical breakdown has begun. The highest temperatures recommended for deep frying are 380 to 390 degrees. Among the sunflower and safflower oils tested by *Consumer Reports*, none had a smoke point below 450 degrees. Olive oils, however, range from 315 to 400 degrees smoke point, depending on the brand. These probably should be avoided for high-temperature cooking. The peanut oils tested did not smoke below 425 degrees, except for Planters brand, which smoked around 400. According to the Canola Council of Canada, canola oil's smoke point rests safely above 445 degrees.

Here's a list of the various vegetable oils on the market today, with their proportions of polyunsaturated, monounsaturated, and saturated fats.

Vegetable Oils Ranging from Lowest to Highest in Saturated Fat

Type of Oil	Percent saturated	Percent polyunsaturated	Percent monounsaturated
Canola (rapeseed)	6	28	62
Almond	8	17	70
Safflower	9	74	12
Walnut Oil	9	63	23
Sunflower	10	66	20
Corn	13	59	24
Olive	14	8	74

Type of Oil	% Saturated	% Polyunsaturated	% Monounsaturated
Sesame	14	42	40
Soy	15	37	43
Peanut	17	32	46
Wheat germ	19	62	15
Cottonseed	26	52	18
Palm	49	9	37
Cocoa butter oil	59	3	33
Palm kernel oil	81	2	11
Coconut oil	87	2	6

(Note: The percentages may not total 100 when added together because of conversion factors from grams of fat to percent of total fat. Source: Food Processor II computer software, ESHA Research.)

Putting the Squeeze on Margarine

Life without butter is a life condemned to butterless popcorn, bread from the oven or a hot baked potato with something else on it. To me, anything BUT butter IS "something else." But then butter and I go way back.

Have you ever been madly disappointed because someone asked you if you would like some "butter," only to realize they really meant "margarine?" Well, I'm sorry, but margarine is not butter. Margarine is margarine. Which brings us to the question, "Is margarine really that much better for you?"

I'm afraid this is one of those "yes, but . . ." answers. Some of you might be blurting out, "Of course, the answer is yes. What could possibly be just cause for a 'but'?"

This may come as a surprise to some committed margarine users, but margarine has just as much fat (and just as many calories) per teaspoon as butter. Both are made up of approximately 80 percent fat and 20 percent water. Both, of course, have all of their calories from fat. Margarine's claim to fame has to do with the fact that it offers less saturated fat and no cholesterol.

So the one "but" to the "Is margarine better for you" question is that some people tend to use "more" margarine because it has less flavor than butter. And if lowering the total amount of fat in your diet is really the most important diet recommendation, then there are times when butter might be better!

What about the saturated fat and cholesterol you get from butter and not margarine? If you're eating a diet low in fat and saturated fat (using table fats sparingly and cooking with almost no added fat), then it's possible the amount of saturated fat and cholesterol you would get from this incidental table butter may not add up to anything worth worrying about.

If the worst thing that could happen is you use one teaspoon of butter a day, we're talking about adding 10 milligrams of cholesterol. (The daily recommendation is to eat less than 300 milligrams.) The one teaspoon of butter adds about 2 1/2 grams of saturated fat to your day's total.

If you're laughing yourself silly over the concept of only one teaspoon a day, then perhaps you're a candidate for the make-it-with-margarine club. Up to 27 percent of margarine's total fat is from saturated fat, compared to butter with 64 percent.

First there were butter substitutes and the product line "margarine" was born. Well, now there are even substitutes for margarine—the "spreads" or "diet margarines." These products basically can't legally be called margarine because they contain less than the federally required 80 percent fat (by weight). Spreads, for example, are usually between 45 and 75 percent fat by weight. How does this 5 to 35 percent fat magically disappear? Food manufacturers not so magically just add more water.

Then there's the "whipped" butter or margarine (where air is incorporated into the product during the whipping process). These products also have less fat per teaspoon. So take your pick. You can replace some of the fat with air or with water. But it only counts (in terms of health) if you use the same amount or less than you would normally.

In case you're in the market for a good tasting margarine, *Consumer Reports* conducted a taste test on the subject a few years ago. The top three were, in this order:

#1. I Can't Believe It's Not Butter (stick)

    (Per tablespoon, 90 calories, 95 mg sodium, and 20% saturated fat)

#2. Parkay (stick)

    (Per tablespoon, 100 calories, 155 mg sodium, 18% saturated fat)

#3. Blue Bonnet

    (Per tablespoon: 100 calories, 95 mg sodium, 18% saturated fat)

But, you need to know that this taste test was done before my favorite margarine was available: It's Dairy Maid Light Spread made by, of all people, the Challenge Butter Company. Their diet margarine is made mostly of water, then butter, then liquid corn oil. One teaspoon has 20 calories, 2 grams of fat, and 1.1 milligrams cholesterol. Of the 2 grams of fat, 1 gram is saturated. I keep hearing there are people who actually prefer the taste of margarine, but I have yet to meet any. Perhaps these top-tasting margarines will make a difference.

You have to make up your own mind. Obviously we all should be using much less fat overall—on the table and in our cooking. If we would add the same amount of either, then a less-saturated margarine would be the spread of choice. But what I find are that margarine users tend to use more margarine, perhaps in an effort to compensate for the lack of flavor.

"Hydrogenation"—A Sign of Saturation

The "hydrogenation" process, commonly used to produce shortening and more solid margarines (from a liquid vegetable oil), actually "saturates" some of an oil's poly- or monounsaturated fats.

This hydrogenation process has also infiltrated the packaged food industry. You'll find it in your crackers, cookies, frozen dairy desserts, etc. You'll find the words "hydrogenated" or "partially hydrogenated vegetable oil" listed on the ingredient label if it's in there.

When an oil is "hydrogenated" or "partially hydrogenated," it undergoes a processing procedure where hydrogen ions are pumped into a vegetable oil, changing some of its "unsaturated fatty acids" (either mono- or polyunsaturated) to newly "saturated fatty acids." Theoretically, the softer, more liquid margarines are less saturated because they need less hydrogenation.

Summing It All Up

Before we wrap up this course in low-fat eating, how about humoring the teacher in me and taking a little quiz? (Ah, come on! It's true or false.)

1. When you eat a Big Mac, you are really swallowing the equivalent in fat grams of 7 teaspoons of oil!

2. A turkey ham, advertised as "95% Fat-Free" can be a high-fat product in disguise (50 percent of its calories may come from fat). The ad phrase "95 percent Fat-Free" really refers to it being 5 percent fat BY WEIGHT, but half of its calories may still be from fat!

3. Thirty percent of ALL CANCERS in this country are thought to be preventable through changes in our DIET.

4. The typical evening party goer, without any extra effort, can walk out of a party having eaten a minimum of 2,200 calories, most of which are from fat.

5. The chef salad that many people often order when they're watching their weight is really one of the fattiest, highest calorie choices they could make (approximately 800 calories each, 72 percent of which are from fat).

6. By making simple changes to a chocolate cake mix, you can bake an irresistible chocolate whiskey cake that has only 200 calories a slice and 22 percent of calories from fat, compared to the usual cake mix recipe with 300 calories a slice and 48 percent of calories from fat.

7. You can cut the fat almost in half in some of the fast food sandwiches, such as the Fillet-O-Fish at McDonald's, just by taking off the mayonnaise, fatty secret sauces, or tartar sauce.

8. Two comprehensive, research-based, government health reports were released to the public recently and both focused on the importance of lowering the fat in the American diet.

9. Cheese and beef aren't necessarily "bad" foods. They CAN be part of a low-fat dish when smaller amounts of the lower-fat options (part-skim cheese and the leanest beef cuts) are eaten, along with complex carbohydrates with a limited amount of fat added.

Did you think all of the statements were TRUE?

Congratulations. If you got most of them right, then you should feel good about what you've learned over the last ten chapters. Which brings me to the final requirement for fighting fat forever—self-confidence. You need to feel as if you fully understand the basic steps to eating a low-fat diet.

Never let down your guard because it really is a "fight" against FAT. Fat wears many different disguises. It comes by way of the kitchen table (from table fats such as butter, margarine, sour cream, gravy, salad dressing) or stove (deep-fat frying, fats added in the pan). We are most often fooled by the "hidden fats," those in foods that protect their presence well, such as crackers (even "baked" wheat thins), frozen waffles, bakery muffins, ice creams, and many others.

I'm having a difficult time ending this book because the road to low-fat eating never really ends. There will always be newly discovered (and delicious) low-fat recipes to share, new products to tell you or warn you about, new fast food items, and new trendy type restaurants to give you tips on. But for now, you definitely know the basics.

And if, per chance, your health and your vigor for low-fat eating change positively because of this book, then please share your enthusiasm (and the title of this book) with someone you love. It could make a big difference in their lives, and in yours.

INDEX

Convenience Food Facts by Arlene Monk, R.D., C.D.E., with an introduction by Marion Franz, R.D., M.S. Includes complete nutrition information, tips, and exchange values on more than 1,500 popular name brand processed foods commonly found in grocery store freezers and shelves. Helps you plan easy-to-prepare, nutritious meals.

004081   ISBN 0-937721-77-8 $10.95   ☐

Fast Food Facts by Marion Franz, R.D., M.S. This revised and up-to-date best-seller shows how to make smart nutrition choices at fast food restaurants–and tells what to avoid. Includes complete nutrition information on more than 1,000 menu offerings from the 21 largest fast food chains.

Standard-size edition 004240   ISBN 1-56561-043-1 $7.95   ☐
Pocket edition 004228   ISBN 1-56561-031-8 $4.95   ☐

The Healthy Eater's Guide to Family & Chain Restaurants by Hope S. Warshaw, M.M.Sc., R.D. Here's the only guide that tells you how to eat healthier in over 100 of America's most popular family and chain restaurants. It offers complete and up-to-date nutrition information and suggests which items to choose and avoid.

004214   ISBN 1-56561-017-2 $9.95   ☐

Exchanges for All Occasions by Marion Franz, R.D., M.S. Exchanges and meal planning suggestions for just about any occasion, sample meal plans, special tips for people with diabetes, and more.

004201   ISBN 1-56561-005-9 $12.95   ☐

366 Low-Fat Brand Name Recipes in Minutes by M. J. Smith, M.A., R.D./L.D. Here's more than a year's worth of the fastest family favorites using the country's most popular brand name foods–from Minute Rice® to Ore Ida®–while reducing unwanted calories, fat, salt and cholesterol.

004247   ISBN 1-56561-050-4 $12.95   ☐

Emergency Medical Treatment: Infants, Children, Adults: Revised and Expanded Edition by Stephen Vogel, M.D., and David Manhoff, produced in cooperation with the National Safety Council. With over 1.5 million copies sold, the #1–selling guide of its kind has saved countless lives and is now totally updated with the newest safety guidelines. Written especially for people untrained in emergency medical procedures, this indispensable, step-by-step guide tells exactly what to do during the most common, life-threatening situations you might encounter for infants, children, and adults.

004627   ₒ   ISBN 0-916363-10-4 $12.95   ☐

Taking the Work Out of Working Out by Charles Roy Schroeder, Ph.D. This motivational book shows you step-by-step ways to turn all forms of exercise–from aerobics to weight lifting–into enjoyable, creative, and sensual experiences that you'll look forward to. With the aid of over 30 photographs, illustrations and charts, beginners and professionals alike can avoid feeling worn-out and improve their workout.

004246   ISBN 1-56561-049-0 $9.95   ☐

All-American Low-Fat Meals in Minutes by M.J. Smith R.D., L.D., M.A. Filled with tantalizing recipes and valuable tips, this cookbook makes great-tasting low-fat foods a snap for holidays, special occasions, or everyday. Most recipes take only minutes to prepare.
004079   ISBN 0-937721-73-5 $12.95

One Year of Healthy, Hearty, and Simple One-Dish Meals by Pam Spaude and Jan Owan-McMenamin, R.D., is a collection of 365 easy-to-make healthy and tasty family favorites and unique creations that are meals in themselves. Most of the dishes take under 30 minutes to prepare.
004217   ISBN 1-56561-019-9 $12.95

200 Kid-Tested Ways to Lower the Fat in Your Child's Favorite Foods by Elaine Moquette-Magee, M.P.H., R.D. For the first time ever, here's a much needed and asked for guide that gives easy, step-by-step instructions on cutting the fat in the most popular brand name and homemade foods kids eat every day–without them even noticing.
004231   ISBN 1-56561-034-2 $12.95

60 Days of Low-Fat, Low-Cost Meals in Minutes by M.J. Smith, R.D., L.D., M.A. Following the path of the best-seller *All American Low-Fat Meals in Minutes,* here are more than 150 quick and sumptuous recipes complete with the latest exchange values and nutrition facts for lowering calories, fat, salt, and cholesterol. This book contains complete menus for 60 days and recipes that use only ingredients found in virtually any grocery store—most for a total cost of less than $10.
004205   ISBN 1-56561-010-5 $12.95

CHRONIMED Publishing
P.O. Box 47945
Minneapolis, MN 55447-9727
Place a check mark next to the book (s) you would like sent. Enclosed is $_____. (Please add $3.00 to this order to cover postage and handling. Minnesota residents add 6.5% sales tax.) Send check or money order, no cash or C.O.D.'s. Prices are subject to change without notice.

Name _____

Address _____

City _____ State _____ Zip _____

Allow 4 to 6 weeks for delivery.
Quantity discounts available upon request.
Or order by phone: 1-800-848-2793,
612-546-1146 (Minneapolis/St. Paul metro area).
Please have your credit card number ready.